The Essential Guide to
Multiple Sclerosis

Robert Duffy Series Editor

Published in Great Britain in 2017 by
need2know
Remus House
Coltsfoot Drive
Peterborough
PE2 9BF
Telephone 01733 898103
www.need2knowbooks.co.uk

Contents

Introduction

This book is a combination of essential information about multiple sclerosis (MS) and first hand experience of living with the condition. Presented in an easy-to-read format, it will equip you with useful tools and coping strategies whether you are newly diagnosed, have lived with MS for years, or perhaps have a friend, family member or colleague with the condition. Crammed with practical advice and the latest medical information, it will lift the lid on some of the preconceptions and mysteries surrounding MS. It covers what MS is, how it develops, the types of MS, treatments available and offers advice about lifestyle changes that can help with symptom management.

Latest statistics from the MS Society indicate that there are 100,000 people with MS in the UK. It is the most common disabling neurological condition affecting young adults – many of them diagnosed in their 20s or 30s. In the UK the chance of developing MS is about 1 in 700. For some people, MS is characterised by periods of relapse and remission, while for others it has a progressive pattern.

MS affects many more people than the 100,000 who are living with it. It affects their children, spouse or partner and extended family as well as friends and colleagues. It can affect people who treat the person – whether for their MS or complications resulting from it. If you are one of these people, this book will help you to understand more about this complex condition.

> People tend to form an image of MS, based mainly on the experiences of someone else who they have known or heard of.

Despite MS being a high profile condition, a recent study carried out by the MS Society showed widespread ignorance amongst the general public about the disease, what its symptoms are and at what age it is usually diagnosed. People tend to form an image of MS, based mainly on the experiences of someone else who they have known or heard of. This is a natural assumption, but likely to be very inaccurate.

There is no denying that MS is a puzzling condition, not only for those affected by it, but for scientists working tirelessly to develop new treatments and health professionals overseeing treatments. Due to its complexity and unpredictability, many misconceptions have evolved around MS over the years. This book contains realistic but positive information that challenges outdated misconceptions.

Today, there is better awareness of chronic conditions such as diabetes and asthma, with more people having a general idea why someone they know needs to inject insulin, or use an inhaler. People now understand about different forms of diabetes: Type 1 and Type 2. A similar sea change in awareness is needed with regard to MS, so that people in the wider population can begin to understand the different types of MS and the day-to-day challenges that living with symptoms can bring.

Just 20 years ago, a diagnosis of MS was frequently associated with a bleak future. There is still much work to be done, particularly with regard to the more progressive types of MS, but the last two decades have been a time of advancement. New diagnostic techniques, improved management of symptoms, access to better information and support from health professionals being just some of the factors leading to a better quality of life for people affected by MS.

Some people with MS appear to have few visible symptoms but live with pain; bladder or bowel problems; chronic fatigue; problems with memory, thought processing and mood. A separate chapter in this book deals with these aspects of MS that are often overlooked.

MS is often diagnosed at an age when people are in the prime of their career and have family and financial commitments, typically people in their 20s to 40s. It is important that they know where to go for help and advice. Knowing which questions to ask and who to ask can be a key part of moving into the future with MS. A separate chapter is included on finances and practical matters.

MS is not a 'one size fits all' condition. It is therefore not possible to include detailed information on every aspect of MS within the remits of this guide, but comprehensive information on all the topics mentioned are available from sources such as the MS Society and MS Trust. Full contact details for these organisations along with many others can be found in the help list at the back of this book.

Treat this guide like a toolbox. Take from it the tools that you find useful for your own MS and try not to focus on symptoms that you haven't experienced – and maybe never will. None of us know what tomorrow may bring and many people with MS become experts at living in the moment.

There is no denying that a diagnosis of MS will mean changes. But with the right treatment, support and advice, you can find your own unique balance between having this chronic condition and having a life.

There is still much work to be done, particularly with regard to the more progressive types of MS, but the last two decades have been a time of advancement.

Disclaimer

This book is for general information on MS, and isn't intended to replace professional medical advice. If you have been diagnosed with MS, you should follow the advice given to you by your GP and other healthcare professionals.

All the information in this book was correct at the time of going to press. National guidelines and recommendations change, so it is important to check with your GP or healthcare professional before acting on any of the information in this book.

Particularly long terms have been abbreviated to their initials throughout the book, please make use of the acronyms page if you find you cannot remember what each one stands for.

With the right treatment, support and advice, you can find your own unique balance between having this chronic condition and having a life.

Acronyms

CCSVI chronic cerebrospinal venous insufficiency

CIS clinically isolated syndrome

CSF cerebrospinal fluid

DDA Disability Discrimination Act

DEA disability employment advisor

DLA Disability Living Allowance

DMD disease modifying drugs

EBV Epstein-Barr virus

EFA essential fatty acid

FES functional electrical stimulation

LDN low dose naltrexone

OCB oligoclonal bands

OT occupational therapist

PML progressive multifocal leukoencephalopathy

TENS transcutaneous nerve stimulation

VER visual evoked response

1

Myths, Facts and Multiple Sclerosis

What the perception used to be

s recently as the 1980s, many people lived with multiple sclerosis (MS) for years without ever knowing the cause of their symptoms.

Few people got the chance to see a neurologist. They received most of their care from their GP, who would have had little or no knowledge of MS.

What happened if you were diagnosed?

Even with a diagnosis, the perception of MS seemed to range somewhere between 'pull yourself together' and 'expect the worst…'.

Common advice given to patients on diagnosis was 'You've got MS – go home and learn to live with it.' This often led to people withdrawing from many activities and waiting for severe physical disability to overtake them. Even if that never happened, they were emotionally and psychologically disabled from the moment of diagnosis.

> In the absence of today's diagnostic techniques, myths about MS were commonplace.

In the absence of today's diagnostic techniques, myths about MS were commonplace. A diagnosis of MS implied that you would 'end up in a wheelchair' at some time, which was not an incentive for a person to stay as active as possible. It was also assumed that MS would place a heavy burden on patients, their families and caregivers, the health system and society. Younger women with MS were even told that they should never have children.

Doctors would not generally recommend exercise due to the perception that it could make a person's MS worse. MS patients were not routinely offered physiotherapy or support and advice. Lack of regular, sensible exercise would have made it difficult to maintain muscle tone, increasing the likelihood of falls. It may have also contributed to low mood and increased fatigue levels.

The importance of good nutrition in managing MS was not understood. As a result of inactivity and poor diet, there was an increased likelihood of people with MS becoming malnourished or overweight, further affecting their quality of life. Frequent bladder infections would perhaps have contributed to a higher relapse rate.

Most care would have been left to family members. Those without family support and increasing disability may have ended up in a hospital or care home – many of them still only in their 40s and 50s.

When did it change?

Changes have happened gradually over the past 50 or so years:

- 1950 – MS was formally recognised as a disease of the central nervous system, putting an end to common misconceptions around it being a mental illness.

- 1953 – the UK MS Society was founded by Richard Cave. Today it has over 350 local branches and some 40,000 members.

- 1972 – Ian MacDonald and Martin Halliday introduced a new diagnostic method. Visually evoked potentials allowed doctors to measure the speed of messages along the optic nerves.

- 1978 – computer tomography (CT) was used in MS diagnosis. This layered X-ray examination method showed the first images of larger MS lesions.

- 1980 – cortisone, an anti-inflammatory hormone, proved to be beneficial in the treatment of MS by speeding up recovery from relapses.

- 1981 – Ian R. Young and Graham M. Bydder revolutionised MS diagnosis by using magnetic resonance imaging. MRI showed up lesions in the brain and allowed the progress of the disease to be followed.

- 1985 – McAlpine's Multiple Sclerosis (second edition) was published (Philadelphia, Churchill Livingstone) by Alistair Compston, Ian McDonald, John Noseworthy and others. It became a standard for health professionals working on the front line with MS and in research.

- 1993 – the MS Trust was founded in the UK by Chris Jones and Jill Holt. The organisation provides information, education, research and support for those affected by MS and for the health professionals responsible for their care.

- 1995 – beta interferon became the first licensed treatment to modify the condition. The MS Trust agreed to take on an educational role and set to work developing the expertise in-house to run an accredited education programme for specialist nurses.

- 2001 – an international group of experts, lead by Ian McDonald, published new and reliable diagnostic criteria that also included MRI findings, meaning suitable patients could start treatment sooner.

How it has changed?

- Diagnosis today is usually made by a neurologist, based on your symptoms and what they find when they examine you, plus results from a range of diagnostic tests.

- People are being diagnosed earlier in the course of their illness. Those who clinicians believe will benefit from treatment now have more time to respond to drugs and treatment, thereby slowing down the disease progression and reducing the possibility of long-term disability.

- People living with MS should now have access to a specialist MS nurse who works alongside neurologists and other specialists. Newly diagnosed MS patients should be offered the chance to attend a series of information sessions with their MS nurse, where they will also meet others facing similar circumstances and learn important self-help strategies.

- Since beta interferon was introduced, several more disease modifying drugs have been licensed for certain types of MS. Most of these treatments are self-injected. MS nurses play a key role in teaching patients how to administer their medication and learning how to deal with possible side effects.

There is still much work to be done, particularly with regard to the more progressive types of MS, but the past 20 years have been a time of achievement. New diagnostic techniques, improved management of symptoms, access to information and support from health professionals being just some of the factors leading to a better quality of life for people affected by MS.

Just as myths of doom and gloom abounded in the past, it is important to watch for more modern myths which can be just as damaging to today's MS community. Many of these are communicated to us via the media.

How do I know what to believe?

Just as myths of doom and gloom abounded in the past, it is important to watch for more modern myths which can be just as damaging to today's MS community. Many of these are communicated to us via the media.

You are most likely to hear about new research in the daily news media, where there is not necessarily space or interest in full references to back up the story. Good journalists usually indicate whether research has been published and mention the name of the scientific journal it has appeared in, but this is not always the case.

The media has been a great help in raising awareness of MS as well as raising funds for research and enabling people within the world wide MS community to link up, exchange and support each other.

For many of those diagnosed today, the Internet will be their first port of call when it comes to finding out about MS and treatments available. It is important to remember though that much of this information is based on other people's opinions and experiences. What has worked for them may indeed help you, but it could also harm you. Always seek advice from a healthcare professional before committing to any form of non-conventional treatment.

Another recent example of imbalanced media coverage resulted in an alarming association with MS and dying. This caused much anguish within the MS community and for their families and friends. Most people with MS will live as long as anyone else, but this was not made clear in the media coverage because it was not the main focus of that particular news story. MS is not a terminal illness.

Case studies

MS prior to the 1990s

'As a teenager in 1956, I had weird symptoms for years, but they suddenly became a lot worse and I was sent to hospital. It was a strange time. I was in a ward with lots of people with the same symptoms as myself and there was a feeling "It's all in the mind." There were loads of doctors crowding around my bed talking about me as if I was an object and I vaguely heard "MS" and then "This one's not likely to reach 25."

'The symptoms lasted for about six months, but I was not told of my diagnosis and I went back to school. My headmaster told me "There's no point buying books for university; I've cancelled your place." He said I was unlikely to reach 25 so there was no point educating me! When I applied for jobs I was told: "There's no point in training you; you'll be dead before you reach 25." I persevered and got a job with a publisher.

'Before we were married, my husband was advised by our GP not to marry me because I wouldn't be able to have children and he'd end up looking after me. Three years later, after we moved house, my husband told me what the GP had said, and it was only then that I finally found out I had MS.

'My new GP admitted to not knowing a lot about MS, so he went on a course and was then able to recognise that MS changes from day-to-day, hour-to-hour. I was hill-walking until 1992 when I had a very bad relapse and had to leave work. I now have an electric scooter with a swivel seat which I garden from. I have one hour of exercise in the morning and again in the evening.' AA (© MS Society, *MS Matters Magazine*).

MS in the 2000s

LP was diagnosed with MS in 2004 aged 19.

'When I left school, I trained in catering and became a chef working long hours and different shifts. One morning when I opened my eyes I found that I couldn't see properly. I ended up in hospital for a week while they did lots of blood tests, a lumbar puncture, CT and MRI scans. I was diagnosed with MS. During the next year, I had several more relapses which affected my eyes and legs as well as nerve pain in one arm and hand.

'My neurologist suggested I take part in a trial for a new drug. I had to go to hospital every so often to be given the treatment via intravenous drip. I felt nauseous for 24 hours after treatment and my hair thinned a bit temporarily. Since beginning the trial two years ago, I haven't had a major relapse. I still experience fatigue and pain but am learning how to manage it and I'm taking one of the disease modifying therapies to help reduce the chances of relapses.

'I decided to change my career path from catering which was physically very demanding to accountancy. I now work in an office and am studying at night school. My employer knows I have MS and has been very supportive.' LP.

Summing Up

- Less than 20 years ago, old myths about MS were commonplace. One of these was that MS meant you would one day end up in a wheelchair.

- The MS Society was set up in 1953. It funds MS research, runs respite care centres and provides grants, education and training on MS. It produces numerous publications on MS and runs a website and freephone specialist helpline. There are over 350 local branches across the UK.

- The 1990s was a key decade, with improved diagnostic techniques giving people with MS better access to advice and symptom management.

- The MS Trust, established in 1993, took on a vital educational role when the first specialist MS nurses were trained not just to help those eligible for new drugs, but to improve care for everyone with MS.

- In 1995, beta interferon became the first licensed treatment to modify the condition rather than treat symptoms.

- Don't believe everything you hear or read about in the media – modern myths can be just as damaging and misleading as the old ones!

2

What is MS?

MS is a condition which affects the central nervous system – the body's control centre for actions, senses and activities. Multiple stands for many. 'Sclerosis' comes from the Greek 'skleros' meaning hard. In MS, hard areas, or scars, develop around the damaged nerves.

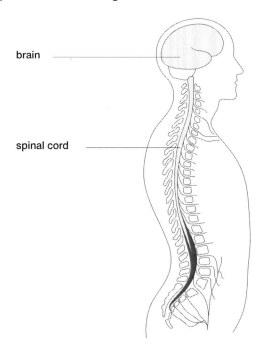

brain

spinal cord

The central nervous system – MS occurs when there is damage to the myelin around the nerves in the central nervous system. The central nervous system is made up of the brain and the spinal cord. (© MS Society, *Just Diagnosed – An Introduction to MS*, 05/09.)

At present there is no cure for MS which means that once it develops it is classed as a lifelong condition.

The first identifiable case of MS was described by Augustus d'Este, a grandson of King George III, about 150 years ago. His MS was recognised from a diary he kept describing his symptoms in. Since then, it has become one of the most common conditions faced by clinical neurologists, as well as one of the most intriguing puzzles for neuroscientists.

What causes MS?

Usually, our immune system protects us from outside attackers like germs and viruses. If we get an infection and our temperature goes up, it means our immune system is doing its job. When someone has an MS relapse, or an 'attack', it is actually caused by the body's own immune system attacking part of their central nervous system. MS is therefore classed as an autoimmune condition.

There are three processes which take place in MS:

- Inflammation: nerves run through the central nervous system carrying messages between the brain and the rest of the body. Each nerve is coated with a substance called 'myelin', which helps to speed up the smooth transfer of messages around the body. In MS, inflammatory cells attack the myelin coating, causing fluid to collect around them which compresses the nerve and prevents messages getting through to parts of the body. When the fluid disappears and no longer compresses the nerve fibres, this is called remission.

- Demyelination: inflammation sometimes causes scars which can damage the myelin coating on a nerve, a process called demyelination. In non-medical terms this could perhaps be described as a 'raw nerve'. Symptoms will vary depending on which nerves are affected and how bad the damage is. Therefore, no two people will have exactly the same combination of symptoms or rate of disease progression.

- Axonal loss: inflammation can also lead to complete severing of a nerve, which means that this part of the nerve will stop functioning and the whole nerve fibre may die; this is called axonal loss.

MS has become one of the most common conditions faced by clinical neurologists, as well as one of the most intriguing puzzles for neuroscientists.

Myelin

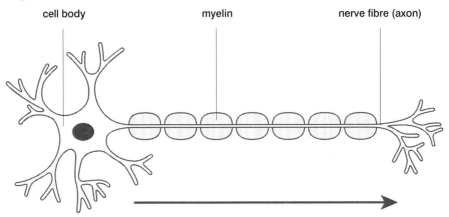

Myelin coats the nerve fibres (axons). Myelin helps the axons in the central nervous system conduct messages. Myelin also protects the axons. (© MS Society, *Just Diagnosed – An Introduction to MS*, 05/09.)

Demyelination in MS

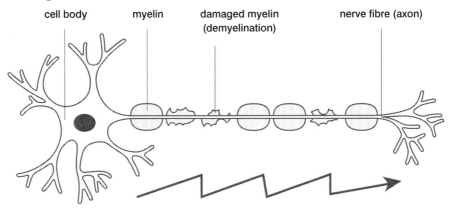

In MS, there is damage to the myelin (demyelination) which can cause messages to be slowed down, distorted or blocked. Messages can also be affected by damage to the nerve fibres themselves. (© MS Society, *Just Diagnosed – An Introduction to MS*, 05/09.)

Most people find all this hard to understand...

The same damage process that can make it difficult for one person to walk, can cause another person to experience double vision or fatigue. This is often hard for people to understand because it all happens inside the body and out of view.

It can help to compare a nerve to an electricity cable – if the plastic coating on a cable is trapped or damaged, leaving the copper wires exposed, power passing through it might be interrupted. There is also a chance that frayed wires might react with each other as in 'crossed wires', making lights flicker on and off. In the same way, when the myelin coating on a nerve becomes scarred, messages can be slowed down, mixed up or blocked.

A reminder of some terms used so far

It can sometimes feel as though MS brings with it a whole new dictionary of words! Here are a few of the ones used so far:

- Multiple stands for many.

- Sclerosis means scarring.

- Inflammation in MS is the swelling that occurs during an attack.

- Demyelination is the stripping of the myelin from the surface of nerves.

- Axonal loss is the death of nerve fibres.

- An autoimmune condition is a disorder of the immune system in which the processes that usually defend against disease attack the body's own tissues.

> The same damage process that can make it difficult for one person to walk, can cause another person to experience double vision or fatigue.

Who gets MS?

Nobody knows exactly why some people get MS and others don't. A huge amount of research is going on to try and find the answers and each year our knowledge is increasing.

Latest estimates (MS Society, 2009) indicate that there are at least 100,000 people living with MS in the UK. It is the most common neurological condition affecting young adults in Western countries and is usually diagnosed in people in their 20s to 40s.

- In the general population in the UK, the risk of developing MS is about 1 in 700.

- MS does not usually begin in childhood and is unlikely to develop in later life, though there is a less common type of progressive MS that can start in people who are in their 40s or 50s.

- It is thought that at least twice as many women as men have MS, with some studies indicating this ratio has risen to 3:1. Researchers are looking into the role hormones may play.

- MS is not infectious – you can't catch it like you can illnesses such as colds or flu, which are caused by bacteria or a virus.

- It is thought that genes play a role, along with possible environmental factors.

- MS is not a terminal illness – most people will live as long as anyone else.

Types of MS

MS can affect a person in a wide variety of ways. The features of the condition are known as symptoms and can vary in location and severity from person to person. Due to advancements in diagnostic techniques and medical knowledge, it is now possible to identify different types of MS.

Why does it matter which type of MS I have?

Health professionals need to know which type of MS you have in order to decide on the best way to treat or manage your condition. With some types of MS, the earlier treatment commences, the more effective it can be in reducing long-term disability.

All MS treatments have to undergo thorough clinical trials before being licensed for use. Not all MS drugs are suitable for all types of MS. Using the results from large-scale clinical trials, doctors are able to determine which people will be likely to benefit the most from which treatment.

If doctors do not believe a type of treatment would make any difference to a person's symptoms, and perhaps cause unwanted side effects, they may decide that it is not ethical or cost effective for them to prescribe it.

How is the type identified?

The type of MS can be identified by looking at:

- The symptoms a person has experienced.
- The way the symptoms have changed over a period of time.
- The results of diagnostic tests carried out.

How many types of MS are there?

There are four main types of MS:

- Relapsing remitting MS.
- Primary progressive MS.
- Secondary progressive MS.
- Progressive relapsing MS.

Relapsing remitting MS

In relapsing remitting MS, once the attack by the immune system has stopped, the myelin is able to repair itself. In some people, the myelin completely repairs itself and symptoms will disappear for a period of time. This is known as a period of remission. Symptoms usually develop over a few days, stabilise over a few weeks and then slowly improve over weeks or months.

Primary progressive MS

In primary progressive MS, the myelin is unable to repair itself right from the start, resulting in earlier permanent damage to the nerves. This is called progression, rather than relapsing. The progression of disability will depend on how often the same nerves are affected. This is the rarest type of MS, involving about 10% of cases.

Secondary progressive MS

In secondary progressive MS, if the same area of myelin is attacked repeatedly by the body's immune system, scar tissue can appear where the myelin has repaired itself, just as it would if we had a scar from an injury or operation. If scarring (or demyelination) happens, permanent damage can be caused to the nerves affected. This is called progression and is what happens when someone's MS changes from relapsing remitting to secondary progressive.

Progressive relapsing MS

In progressive relapsing MS, part of the myelin dies as a result of early attacks by the immune system, but part manages to repair itself, resulting in a possible reduction of some symptoms in the short term. Subsequent attacks to the same nerves will eventually mean that the myelin cannot continue to repair itself, and the damage to the nerves will be permanent. This is called axonal loss.

Other terms sometimes used to describe MS

- Clinically isolated syndrome (CIS) is a fairly new term used to describe someone who has only had one neurological episode or relapse, lasting at least 24 hours. Not everyone who experiences a CIS will go on to develop MS.

- Rapidly evolving MS is another new term used by clinicians to identify a subgroup of people with relapsing remitting MS who they believe will benefit from treatment with a new drug called natalizumab (Tysabri). Further information about new treatments can be found in chapter 10.

- Benign MS is a term used to describe a person who has few relapses and remissions with very good or complete recovery and no accumulation of disability over time as a result of relapses. Many doctors are wary of using this term, as MS can only truly be termed benign if a person has little disability several decades after being diagnosed.

- Malignant MS is used to describe a very aggressive version of the disease where disability accumulates rapidly as a consequence of relapses and/or progression. The use of the term does not imply the condition is cancerous in nature – it is not.

It is important to realise in the early stages of the condition that your doctor may be uncertain about the exact type of MS you have, or indeed whether you have MS at all. A more certain diagnosis may be possible with further investigations and observing how your condition changes over time.

What is meant by the 'course' of MS?

The course of MS is the way it changes or is expected to change over time. It is also referred to by doctors as the 'prognosis' and varies from person to person. Some people with relapsing remitting MS may have very few relapses and complete recovery, whereas others may have frequent relapses with incomplete recovery and accumulate disability as a consequence.

It is impossible to predict the future accurately for an individual person, but researchers have been able to develop some statistics based on an average group of people with MS:

- Approximately 90% of people experience relapses and remissions early in the course of their condition, with the remaining 10% experiencing progression from the onset.

- Most people diagnosed with MS will not need to use a wheelchair on a regular basis.

- On average, approximately half of those with relapsing remitting MS may go on to develop secondary progressive MS after 20 years.

- Developing MS at a younger age is associated with slower accumulation of disability over time.

- Visual or sensory symptoms at onset, good recovery from early relapses, and long gaps between first and second relapses may indicate a slightly better long-term prognosis.

Most people diagnosed with MS will not need to use a wheelchair on a regular basis.

Summing Up

- Nobody knows exactly why some people get MS and others don't. A huge amount of research is going on to try to find the answers.

- MS is a condition of the central nervous system – the brain and spinal cord. Messages to the rest of the body are slowed down and sometimes sent to the wrong place as can happen with faulty electrical wiring.

- MS is an autoimmune condition whereby damage is caused by the body's own immune system mistakenly attacking the myelin coating found on nerves. Sometimes the myelin is able to repair itself, but scar tissue can appear and cause permanent damage over time.

- Symptoms of MS will vary depending on which nerves are affected and how bad the damage is. This means no two people will have exactly the same symptoms or rate of disease progression.

- There are four main types of MS, but even with modern diagnostic techniques it is not always easy for doctors to make a specific diagnosis about the type of MS until time has elapsed.

- The course of MS is the way it changes or is expected to change over time. It is also referred to as the prognosis and varies from person to person.

3

Why Me?

f you have been diagnosed with MS, there will be many questions going through your mind. Could it be something I have brought upon myself? Is it hereditary? Has it been caused by an illness or a stressful experience? These are just some of the questions you may think of – more than likely just after you have left the consultation with your neurologist!

Is it my fault?

Most people diagnosed with MS wonder if there is something they have done that might have triggered it. This is a normal reaction and part of coming to terms with diagnosis. Because MS is such a complicated condition, doctors cannot really answer this question. They know that some people are more at risk of getting MS, but cannot accurately predict who will develop it or why.

It is important to discuss any feelings of guilt or blame that you may have in connection with your MS. Just talking to a close friend, partner or relative about your concerns should help. If it doesn't, your GP or MS nurse may be able to refer you to a counsellor, although provision for counselling through the NHS varies greatly across the UK. The help list at the back of this book gives details of many useful organisations including the MS Society and MS Trust.

It is important to note that it is not the MS itself that is passed down, but only the risk.

Studies by Sadovnick and colleagues (1993) have shown that the likelihood of developing MS is influenced by a combination of a 'genetic predisposition' and an 'environmental trigger'.

What is a genetic predisposition?

Genetic predisposition is a term you may hear a lot in connection with MS. It sounds like a complicated phrase, but put simply it means that a very small risk of developing MS is passed down through the generations. It is important to note that it is not the MS itself that is passed down, but only the risk.

Due to extensive research, a lot more is now known about the role that genes play in MS and they are estimated as contributing 30-35% of the risk factor.

Although the cause of MS is unknown, these studies have enabled scientists to begin to piece together the complex MS jigsaw. Here are a few of the statistics obtained:

- Recent studies suggest that about three times as many women as men have MS.

- An identical twin of a person with MS has a 1 in 4 chance of having or developing MS themselves, whereas a non-identical twin has only a 1 in 50 chance.

- People of different ethnic origins have very different risks of developing MS, regardless of where they now live.

- It is rare to find family groups where several people have MS, but it can happen.

Will my children get MS?

MS is not inherited in the way that the colour of your eyes is passed down through the genes. However, it is now generally accepted that if there is MS in the family, you are more likely to have a genetic predisposition to MS than someone who does not have MS in their family.

- Blood tests are not accurate in predicting risk and genetic counselling is therefore not considered to be particularly useful for people with MS.

Here are some useful statistics obtained from research studies (Compston et al., 2005; Sadovnick et al., 1993, see bibliography):

- Due to the genetic predisposition described above, the child of a parent with MS has a small, increased risk of getting MS compared to the general population where the risk is 1 in 700.

- It is by no means certain that the children of a person with MS will develop MS. In fact, studies have shown that 49 out of 50 children with an affected parent will not go on to develop MS.

- Studies with identical twins have shown us that even when two people share exactly the same genes they will not necessarily both develop MS.

- If you have stepchildren or adopted children, they are no more likely to get MS than someone in the general population, even though they may share the same diet, lifestyle and climate.

What is an environmental trigger?

When scientists talk about our environment, they are not just referring to the part of the world that we live in and the air that we breathe. Our individual environment is also created by our diet and lifestyle and any illness or trauma our bodies may have to deal with.

An environmental trigger can be any combination of where we live, how we live and what happens to us during our lives. It is thought that an environmental trigger might contribute 65-70% of the risk factor of developing MS.

The immune system plays a key role in MS, so it is therefore important to take part in regular, sensible exercise, get adequate sleep and allow time for relaxation.

Why might where we live make a difference?

- MS seems to be more common the further away from the equator that people live.

- Even within in the UK, MS is more common in Scotland, particularly the Shetland Islands and Orkney, where the ratio to the general population is 1 in 500.

- In the USA, MS is more common in the northern and western states than in central or southern ones.

- Research is taking place to determine whether higher rates of sunlight exposure may help to protect people from developing MS by increasing vitamin D levels in the body.

- Studies are also looking into the genetic differences between people in different regions – people of Celtic or Scandinavian ancestry seem to be at greater risk of developing MS.

Why might how we live make a difference?

The other part of our environment is made up of our home and work life and how we spend our leisure time – our lifestyle.

Studies of family groups have not found any evidence to suggest that a shared environment or similarities in lifestyles between family members causes an increased risk of MS (Sadovnick et al.,1993).

Work/life balance

If your work/life balance is not right and you don't look after your body, your immune system may become depleted. The immune system plays a key role in MS, so it is therefore important to take part in regular, sensible exercise, get adequate sleep and allow time for relaxation.

Diet and nutrition

Scientists are investigating the part nutrition may play in both the causes and management of MS. What we do know is that the immune system, which plays a key role in MS, is very sensitive to changes in nutrition.

There are theories about the beneficial effects of a diet low in saturated fat and rich in polyunsaturated fats. One report by Swank and Dugan (see bibliography) followed people on such a diet over 30 years and found no deterioration in MS symptoms, but because the study was uncontrolled some scientists argue that we cannot rely on the results.

> It is important to remember that MS is not an infectious disease and cannot be caught from other people.

The link between MS and diet has not been proven, but it is generally accepted that people with MS are well advised to follow a balanced, healthy diet. Some people find that dietary modification, in terms of taking specific supplements or avoiding particular foods, can be helpful.

Could illness or injury increase my chances of getting MS?

A number of viruses have been investigated over the years, including measles, rubella and a herpes virus HHV-6. The bacterium Chlamydia pneumoniae has also been suggested as a possible cause of MS. It has not been possible to make any definite conclusions with the evidence gathered so far.

Studies carried out by Dr Brenda Banwell, associate professor of paediatrics (neurology) at the Hospital of Sick Children in Toronto, have indicated that there may be a link to certain infections as a trigger for MS. One of these infections is the Epstein-Barr virus (EBV) which can cause glandular fever, but it has been difficult to prove a link as this EBV is present in almost all adults, whether they have MS or not. However, studies in children have revealed different statistics:

- Of the children in the studies without MS, only 40% were found to have been exposed to the EBV virus.

- Of the children in the studies with MS, between 85 to 90% were found to have been exposed to the EBV virus.

Although these findings are interesting, it is important to remember that most people who are infected by these viruses will never develop MS. At present the studies only tell us that infections may be one of a number of factors that interact in ways we do not yet understand to trigger the development of MS.

It is important to remember that MS is not an infectious disease and cannot be caught from other people.

People sometimes wonder if a life event, such as a loss, bereavement or particularly stressful time in your home or work life, may have triggered the onset of MS. Although this may seem to make sense to you when you think back, there is at present no scientific evidence to back this up.

Summing Up

- Having MS is not your fault! It is important to discuss any feelings of guilt or blame that you may have in connection with your MS with a member of your family, a friend or a health professional.

- Studies have shown that the likelihood of developing MS is influenced by a combination of a genetic predisposition (35%) and an environmental trigger (65-70%).

- It is not the MS itself that is passed down through generations, but only the small risk. This is what is meant by a genetic predisposition.

- It is by no means certain that the children of a person with MS will develop MS. In fact, studies have shown that 49 out of 50 children of an affected parent will not go on to develop MS.

- The immune system plays a key role in MS, so it is therefore important to take part in regular, sensible exercise, get adequate sleep and allow time for relaxation.

- The link between MS and diet has not been proven, but it is generally accepted that people with MS are well advised to follow a balanced, healthy diet.

- It is important to remember that MS is not an infectious disease and cannot be caught from other people.

- Despite the many theories and personal stories you may hear, there is at present no scientific evidence to prove that a stressful life event or injury can itself be a trigger for MS.

4

Testing for MS

The thought of diagnostic tests can be alarming if you have previously had little or no regular contact with the health system. It can conjure up many different images, depending on your own life experiences.

Although you may be anxious to understand what is causing these mysterious symptoms you have been experiencing, getting a diagnosis of MS can be a long and difficult process. This is not least because the symptoms of MS are common to many other conditions and are likely to come and go if the central nervous system repairs itself, or re-routes messages via different pathways in order to avoid damaged areas.

This chapter provides information about the tests used to diagnose MS and why they are necessary, in easy-to-understand terms that will help you to feel less intimidated by some of the medical jargon you may hear during the diagnostic process.

Neurologists often prefer to wait for a second relapse or for symptoms to become more severe before giving a definite diagnosis.

The steps to diagnosis

The symptoms experienced in MS depend on the position and extent of the scarring or lesions within the central nervous system and on how much damage has occurred, so no two people with MS will have exactly the same set of symptoms.

For these reasons and others, neurologists often prefer to wait for a second relapse or for symptoms to become more severe before giving a definite diagnosis of something that is a lifetime condition – and which at present has no cure.

Common symptoms at the time of diagnosis can include a combination of any of the following:

- Fatigue and concentration problems.
- Loss of vision in one eye.
- Blurred or double vision.
- Dragging a foot.
- Weakness in limbs.
- Reduced co-ordination.
- Balance problems.
- Numbness, pins and needles, burning sensations.

Before making a diagnosis of MS, consultant neurologists will weigh up all of the information they have about your symptoms (what you have told them) along with your medical history, and may also arrange for you to attend various diagnostic tests to give them further information.

What happens next?

In chapter 1, we mentioned how much progress has been made with diagnostic techniques in the past 20 years.

The criteria, or standard currently used by most clinicians to diagnose MS, are called the Revised McDonald Criteria – named after Professor Ian McDonald, the chairman of the original group of MS experts who published their guidelines for diagnosis of MS in 2001. These were revised in 2006.

However, it is important to remember that MS is a very complex condition and, even now, the tests do not always give a definitive result. A misdiagnosis of MS can be very damaging, so be assured that any tests you are required to attend will be essential in providing the best evidence on which to make a correct diagnosis.

Appointments before diagnosis

The first time you meet your neurologist they will want to find out about your clinical history. This is based on what you tell your doctor about your medical history and symptoms, usually supported by some simple physical examinations.

During an appointment in a busy hospital clinic, it is not always easy to remember symptoms you may have experienced some time ago. Symptoms of MS can also include problems with memory and thinking which can feel worse under pressure. Later in this book you will find advice on how to make the best use of your appointments with health professionals, e.g. preparing in advance and possibly taking either a family member or friend with you.

You may have been living with different symptoms for a while. If these symptoms are unpredictable and on the whole invisible to others, you may sometimes feel that nobody believes you. But it is important to remember that health professionals will be keen to listen to what you have to say as it will help them to either rule out or confirm certain aspects and decide whether future tests are appropriate.

MRI scanning

What happens at an MRI scan?

Magnetic resonance imaging (MRI) scans are carried out by a radiographer, who will run through a list of questions before you have the scan to make sure it is safe. This is because MRI scans involve magnetic fields.

- You will be asked to remove any metal objects, including jewellery, piercings, watches and credit cards.

- If there is any chance that you are pregnant, you should inform your doctor or radiographer beforehand and the scan will normally take place after the birth.

- You cannot usually have an MRI scan if you have a pacemaker or cochlear (ear) implant as the magnetic field will interfere with their function.

- Always speak to your doctor or radiographer before the scan if you have any concerns.

- You will be asked to lie very still for 10-15 minutes while the scanner is in operation and will hear a lot of loud banging and clicking noises. You can't take anyone in with you, but you can ask the radiographer to talk to you via headphones or ask for music to help you relax.

- Relaxation techniques including visualisation can be helpful during an MRI scan if you have used them at other times and found them to be beneficial.

- If you are very nervous, you may arrange with your doctor for a sedative to be given beforehand, but you will not be allowed to drive afterwards.

It is important to remember that health professionals will be keen to listen to what you have to say.

What does an MRI scan show?

- An MRI scan can detect areas of inflammation in the brain or spinal cord known as 'white matter'. The inflammation shows as white dots, or lesions, against a grey background.

- A neurologist will be able to study the scan and the number, size and position of these white dots. Using the combined results of various tests, they will decide whether or not the abnormalities are consistent with a diagnosis of MS.

It is difficult to understand what is going on inside us. If we cut a finger, we can see and feel the damage straightaway, even the smallest paper cut. It might help to imagine that an MRI scan is like a photograph which will help your doctors to detect what is happening inside you and put a name to the strange symptoms you may have been experiencing.

For many people, the results of an MRI scan can be a relief, especially if they have experienced a lack of understanding from those around them. Sometimes, the uncertainty can feel worse than the reality.

Areas of the brain commonly affected by MS are: the brainstem, which connects the spinal cord to the main substance of the brain; the cerebellum, which is involved in co-ordination and balance; and the corpus callosum, which contains nerve fibres connecting the left side of the brain to the right.

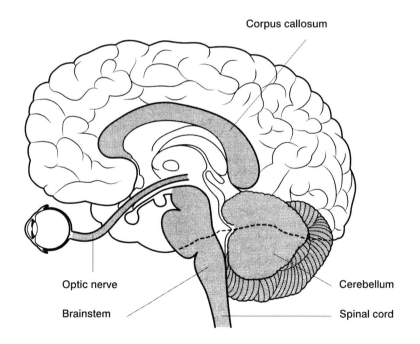

Corpus callosum

Optic nerve

Brainstem

Cerebellum

Spinal cord

Sometimes, the uncertainty can feel worse than the reality.

A midline view of the brain – areas of the brain commonly affected by MS. (© Class Publishing, Multiple Sclerosis – Answers at Your Fingertips, 2009).

With MRI techniques becoming more advanced all the time, damage can be detected in areas of the brain which would previously have appeared as unaffected by MS.

Sometimes a neurologist may suggest that a dye called gadolinium be injected into a vein in your arm before an MRI scan. This can show if there is a fault in the barrier between the circulatory system and the brain, whether areas of inflammation are acute and if they occurred fairly recently.

Lesions in the brain can also occur as part of the normal ageing process, as well as in people with high blood pressure. For these reasons, it is sometimes necessary for people over the age of 50 to have an MRI of the spinal cord as part of the diagnostic process for MS.

It is important to note that for most people with MS, an MRI scan will show some lesions or areas of inflammation, but a small proportion of people with MS have a 'silent' MRI showing none of these factors.

Evoked potentials

Also referred to as visual evoked response (VER), these are simple electrical tests carried out on your vision which can detect a delay in messages between the eyes and the brain. This usually involves an eye test, where you sit in front of a chequer board on a television screen with a number of electrodes attached to your head. It is not a painful procedure.

Because the lagging around the nerves becomes damaged in MS, the electrical nerve impulses travel slower along the nerves and these tests can demonstrate this. It is important to remember that this test is not conclusive on its own and that any abnormalities shown may not necessarily be due to MS.

Lumbar puncture

This procedure, also known as cerebrospinal fluid (CSF) examination, involves drawing a sample of fluid from around the spine and testing for abnormalities that can indicate MS.

A lumbar puncture is usually performed as a day case and it is advisable to arrange for someone to drop you off and pick you up. Your hospital should be able to give you an information sheet about the procedure.

After a lumbar puncture you may have some backache or a headache. It is recommended that you lie flat for a while, drink plenty of fluids and rest for the remainder of the day if you feel you need to.

What happens once the fluid has been removed?

- The spinal fluid is tested for any presence of infection, protein content, sugar levels and a count is taken of the numbers of white and red blood cells in the spinal fluid. It is also tested for the presence of oligoclonal bands (OCBs).

- OCBs are types of proteins that are made by the immune system in response to a trigger. By comparing your spinal fluid and blood, it is possible to see whether the OCBs are only present in the spinal fluid. This would indicate that the immune system has been activated in the brain and/or spinal cord.

- The presence of OCBs is only one aspect of the overall picture considered by your neurologist when making a diagnosis of MS and it is important to note that around 5% of people with definite MS will have a negative lumbar puncture result.

Around 5% of people with definite MS will have a negative lumbar puncture result.

Conditions sometimes confused with MS

If you have been scouring the Internet, the likelihood is you may have discovered many other conditions with symptoms that can be confused with those of MS, including:

- Lupus – lupus or systemic lupus erythomatosis (SLE) is another autoimmune condition that can affect the nervous system, but it also causes skin, joint and kidney problems. Occasionally, people with lupus will have neurological problems that are similar to those seen in MS, but it is unusual for the two conditions to be confused.

- Hughes syndrome – Hughes syndrome or antiphospholipid (AL) syndrome can lead to blood clots in arteries and veins and can sometimes be considered as a potential mimic of MS. Blood tests are used to distinguish between the conditions. In the vast majority of cases, there should be no confusion between Hughes syndrome and MS if a detailed assessment has been undertaken.

- Devic's disease – Devic's disease or neuromyelitis optica (NMO) is a potential MS mimic that causes repeated relapses affecting either the optic (eye) nerves or spinal cord. However, the relapses in Devic's disease are a different sort to those encountered in MS and are usually much more severe, with recovery being incomplete. Blood tests, MRI scanning and lumbar puncture are used to differentiate between Devic's disease and MS.

Summing Up

- The thought of diagnostic tests can be alarming if you've previously had little or no regular contact with the health system. It might conjure up many different images, depending on your own life experiences.

- It is important to remember that health professionals will be keen to listen to what you have to say as it will help them to either rule out or confirm certain aspects and decide whether future tests are appropriate.

- Neurologists often prefer to wait for a second relapse or for symptoms to become more serious before giving a definite diagnosis.

- There are a number of tests used to diagnose MS, including MRI, lumbar puncture and VER. MS is a very complex condition and even now the tests do not always give a definitive result.

- The path to diagnosis can be a long and difficult process, not least because there are other conditions sometimes confused with MS.

5

Diagnosis

verybody with MS has their own diagnosis story, some more complicated than others. It can never be easy for health professionals to deliver a diagnosis affecting a person's life, but the approach that they use can make a huge difference to a person's coping style in both the short and longer term.

This chapter provides information on common issues faced around the time of diagnosis to help you know what to expect and to make the best use of your appointment time.

The consultation

At the neurology clinic

Try to remember that by attending this appointment, you are a step nearer to finding the cause of the mysterious and frustrating symptoms.

Allow yourself plenty of time before your appointment so that you are not arriving in a last minute rush. A neurology clinic in a busy hospital can be a stressful environment, especially if you are unfamiliar with hospitals or have had previous experiences of them which might trigger difficult memories.

It can also feel quite daunting if there are people in the waiting area who need to use mobility equipment in order to get around. It's important that you don't compare yourself to any of the other patients waiting for appointments; a neurology clinic treats a wide variety of neurological conditions as well as MS. Try to remember that by attending this appointment, you are a step nearer to finding the cause of the mysterious and frustrating symptoms that may have been affecting your life for some time.

Many people find it helpful to take a family member or friend with them to their appointment. It is also a good idea to take pen and paper and jot down any questions you may have.

At the appointment with your neurologist

First and foremost, it is important to remember that your consultation is a two way meeting. You must try not to feel anxious about asking questions or seeking clarification from your doctor. There is no right way to react to a diagnosis.

It is quite common for neurologists to use terms like 'probably' when making a diagnosis of MS. This might seem a strange word to use, but MS can be a strange and unpredictable condition. It may be that some of the tests carried out have not given consistent results but, based on all the other information held, the most likely conclusion is MS.

Unlike many other chronic conditions, MS doesn't follow a set pattern. Do not be surprised if your consultant chooses not to go into detail about the many and varied symptoms of MS – you may never experience most of them. However, if the appointment seems hurried and you leave without sufficient information, you could end up struggling on with a symptom without realising that it's connected with your MS, or blame your MS for illnesses which have a completely different cause. So, make sure you ask questions if you have any concerns or need further information.

It is important that your neurologist and other health professionals are made aware of your personal circumstances, including employment, so that you can access the right support and advice for your own MS.

It is important that your neurologist and other health professionals are made aware of your personal circumstances, including employment, so that you can access the right support and advice for your own MS.

Will I be offered any treatment for my MS?

Depending on your prognosis (how your illness is likely to develop), your doctor may also use this consultation to discuss the various drug therapies which are now an established part of managing MS. Information about these is supplied in chapters 9 and 10. They fall into three main groups:

- Drugs to treat relapses.

- Drugs that modify the disease course.

- Drugs to treat symptoms.

Before you leave the consultation, make sure you ask who you should get in touch with regarding the different aspects of your MS and how best to contact them. If you have not already been given details of your nearest MS nurse, do not be frightened to ask. Ask for these contact details in writing, or note them down yourself if you have pen and paper – you may have a lot of information to absorb and it will be difficult to remember everything.

Who will be at the consultation?

Do not be surprised if there are other professionals in the room at your consultation. Many neurology clinics have what is called a multidisciplinary team made up of health professionals involved in the care of patients.

The consultation is likely to include:

- Specialist neurologist – the neurologist is involved in the diagnostic procedure and in determining what medical treatment may be appropriate. A list of specialist MS centres in the UK and the neurologists within those centres can be found on the MS Trust website www.mstrust.org.uk/information/centres.jsp.

- Specialist MS nurse – MS nurses are often the first point of contact to discuss any MS-related concerns. They liaise with, and can refer to, other members of the multidisciplinary team, ensuring continuity of care.

Reactions to diagnosis

A diagnosis of MS generates a wide range of reactions. For some, the shock is profound, sparking a grieving process that takes a long time to come to terms with. For others who may have been worried that they were imagining their symptoms, it can bring tears of relief. Most people will have a reaction that is somewhere in between these two extremes. It is normal for you or those around you to feel any combination of the following initial reactions:

- Anxiety.
- Relief.
- Isolation.
- Sadness.
- Confusion.
- Panic.
- Optimism.
- Fear.
- Denial.
- Hope.

- Shock.

- Anger.

In the days and weeks after diagnosis, it is also natural to have many questions and reactions. If you have to rush back to work or have family commitments after your appointment, it will be normal to push the diagnosis to the back of your mind. If your previous symptoms ease or disappear by the time you receive your diagnosis, it can make the whole situation feel unreal until you experience new symptoms or a recurrence of old symptoms.

If your mind goes blank when the doctor gives you your test results, you might miss the chance to ask several questions. For most MS patients, the best initial point of contact with such questions is your MS nurse, though there are some parts of the UK where there is a shortage of MS nurses. You may need to contact your neurologist through their secretary, or through a referral from your GP if you do not have an MS nurse.

How will MS affect me?

Firstly, it is important to remember that you are the same person before and after diagnosis, with all the same qualities, life skills and experiences. Over time, MS may require you to make adjustments to how you approach different aspects of your life, but just as you yourself are unique, so is your MS.

No one can be certain how MS will affect you. You will hear many new medical terms after your diagnosis, one of which is prognosis. This is simply a term used by doctors to describe how an illness is likely to develop. By reaching a prognosis, doctors can move forward and make decisions as to the best treatment for you as an individual with MS.

Many doctors agree that the first five to seven years of MS can be a good predictor of your future prognosis. Many predictions for MS are based on averages across many people but, as with any average, people can be on either side of this 'average experience' – the average does not always accurately reflect the experiences of an individual.

MS might not yet have a cure, but many people with MS become experts at living in the present moment, finding a new sense of appreciation in many things.

You are the same person before and after diagnosis, with all the same qualities, life skills and experiences.

What can I do to help myself?

There are many things that you can do to help yourself and these might change at different times. Taking care of your body will help you to feel healthier, so exercise and diet are important. Your emotional health is also very important to living with MS. Strong links have been discovered in the past few years between emotions and health. Further information on these topics can be found in chapter 14.

Opportunities to learn more

You may be invited to a course for people with a new diagnosis of MS, where you will have the opportunity to share your experiences with others who are in the same situation. Some people find the thought of attending something like this quite daunting and try to deal with their MS privately, but the feedback from these courses has been overwhelmingly positive.

It cannot be stressed enough that knowing how you can help yourself, as well as knowing where to find help and support from others when you need it, is crucial to living well with MS – both emotionally and physically.

Knowing how you can help yourself, as well as knowing where to find help and support from others when you need it, is crucial to living well with MS.

Learning about your condition and how to manage it can also be a form of self help. You might do this through reading, going to MS Society information days, watching awareness talks on the MS Society or MS Trust websites, or attending an Expert Patient Programme (see help list).

Who should I tell?

There is no rule to follow with this. Some people want to tell everyone, especially if they have been unwell for a time with no apparent reason.

Others prefer to keep it a secret, telling people only on a need to know basis. Sometimes, talking about your diagnosis can be a way of lessening the sense of feeling alone with your MS and of gaining support from others.

If you have a driving licence you must tell the DVLA (Driver and Vehicle Licensing Agency) that you have MS. Chapter 13 gives further information about this along with other official declarations such as those for insurance and employment.

Case study

'I was diagnosed nine years ago. The consultant told me that the tests showed I "probably" had MS, but I wasn't offered any ongoing support or information. He didn't ask what I did for a job or about my family circumstances – my children were small at the time – and made no mention of fatigue or cognitive problems.

'I went straight back to the office afterwards and tried to carry on as normal until my next relapse a few months later. If I'd been given more support and information at diagnosis it would have saved me so many months imagining that I was gong mad – I didn't know that cognitive problems could be part of MS!

'I found out about the MS nurses through the local MS Society branch and went on a course about living well with MS – it made a huge difference. Through a combination of medication and changes to my lifestyle I have learnt how to live positively with MS and take one day at a time.' MM aged 46.

The most effective way to ensure the value of the future is to confront the present courageously and constructively. For the future is born out of, and made by, the present.

Rollo May (author of *Man's Search for Himself*).

Summing Up

- The approach used by health professionals at the point of diagnosis can make a significant difference to the way a person adjusts to living with MS.

- It is best to prepare in advance for the consultation with your neurologist – on the day there will be a lot to take in.

- Remember that your consultation is a two way meeting – ask the questions that you need answers for, and also for the details of who to contact afterwards.

- There is no right way to react to a diagnosis of MS. It is normal to feel many different emotions which will change as time passes.

- There are many things you can do to help yourself – from learning how to take care of your body and emotional health, to sharing and learning with others who are going through similar experiences.

- There are no rules about telling family, friends and colleagues, but talking about your diagnosis to someone close can be a way of lessening your sense of feeling alone.

6

The More 'Visible' Side of MS

S ociety places a great deal of emphasis on the visual image, and the images frequently associated with MS are therefore those that are most visible. This can lead to a 'one size fits all' impression of an illness, based only on people with MS whom we have seen or heard about.

MS, perhaps more than most chronic conditions, is impossible to put in a neat box with a label on. It can be an elusive, unpredictable condition not least in terms of its combination of symptoms and rate of progression. The people it affects come from every conceivable type of background, ranging in age from children to pensioners – all with different coping styles and support networks.

For all the above reasons, this book groups the symptoms of MS in terms of general perception, and therefore the perception commonly held by people before they are diagnosed and go on to learn more about MS.

Not everyone will experience the same symptoms, or experience them with the same frequency or severity.

This chapter describes the more visible symptoms that might be experienced in MS, including those that can affect mobility, speech and tremor, with the next two chapters dealing with symptoms that are perhaps less visible but often just as challenging to live with.

It is important to note that not everyone will experience the same symptoms, or experience them with the same frequency or severity.

Problems with moving and walking

For many people, the image that springs to mind when they hear the words 'multiple sclerosis' is a wheelchair. In reality, most people diagnosed with MS will not need to use a wheelchair on a regular basis.

It is true that some people will develop walking difficulties within 20 years from the start of their condition, but statistics have shown that about 50% of people with relapsing remitting MS will still be walking without mobility aids at that time. Many of them will never need help with walking during their lifetime.

How does MS affect mobility?

Earlier in this book we looked at the causes of MS, along with types, symptoms and the course of the disease. We compared nerves running through the central nervous system to cables carrying electricity, and explained how MS inflammation leaves scars which can damage the surface, resulting in messages being delayed, misdirected or stopped. Difficulties with mobility are caused by this same process.

If you are affected by mobility problems, it is important that the right advice and treatment is obtained at an early stage along with advice on self-help strategies, enabling you to maximise mobility.

Cramps, muscle stiffness and weakness

If a person experiences weak legs and walking difficulties in MS, this could be due to inflammation of the spinal cord. This can cause damage to nerve pathways travelling from their brain to the muscles in their trunk, arms and legs.

If damaged nerves become oversensitive and misfire, it can cause stiffness, cramps and painful spasms where several muscles are contracting at the same time. This is called 'spasticity' and is a common problem in MS. It is important that help is sought as early as possible in order to minimise longer-term problems.

What can help?

A multidisciplinary team of health professionals are needed to manage these aspects of MS and input from a physiotherapist is very important. If you suffer from these problems, treatments may include the following:

- Stretching exercises to maintain muscle flexibility and elasticity.

- Resistance exercises to help increase muscle strength.

- Motion exercises to improve joint movements, reduce joint stiffness and tendon and ligament problems.

- Regular exercise such as swimming to improve overall fitness.

- Drug treatments such as baclofen (Lioresal) to relax the muscles.

It is important that the right advice and treatment is obtained at an early stage along with advice on self help strategies, which can enable a person to maximise their mobility.

Balance, co-ordination and dizziness

If you experience vertigo (spinning sensation), clumsiness or unsteadiness, you may be experiencing inflammation in the brainstem. This is the part of the brain that controls balance and co-ordination.

Dizziness and unsteadiness are common problems with MS and can cause embarrassment in social situations. They are unfortunately difficult to treat and tend not to respond to medications. Spinning sensations can be hard to cope with, but will usually improve over weeks or months.

Eyesight problems

Problems with eyesight can be another sign of inflammation in the brainstem. Visual problems are common in MS and for some people they may be one of the first signs of the condition. They usually get better over days or weeks, although some people do go on to have longer-term problems.

Double vision

When the nerve connections involved in the control of the eye muscles are affected, both eyes may fail to move in unison. If this happens, images will not be aligned correctly, resulting in double vision. If double vision has come on recently, an eye patch may be used as a short-term measure (depending on recovery). If it continues for many weeks or months, a referral to an eye specialist may be needed.

'Jumping' vision

Similarly, damage to the nerve connections can also cause wobbly vision. If the eyes bob up and down or from side to side, it is called 'nystagmus'. If this problem becomes longstanding, it can be very difficult to treat.

Blurred vision and eye pain

Problems with reduced vision or pain, usually in one eye, may result from inflammation of the optic nerve. This is called 'optic neuritis', and is a common problem in people with MS.

The optic nerve carries visual information from the retina, at the back of the eye, to the brain. If you suffer from this, you are likely to notice a blurring of vision in one eye and colours may be less vivid, looking rather grey and washed out. There may also be pain in or behind the eye which is worsened by eye movement.

There is usually good recovery from optic neuritis within a couple of months, but if your vision is affected by your MS, it is likely to be particularly sensitive to your general health and mood. Many people comment that their vision deteriorates when they are tired, stressed or unwell, and if problems persist you should discuss this with your MS nurse or neurologist.

Tremor

Tremor in people with MS is most likely to affect the arms and is usually due to damage to a part of the brain called the cerebellum, or its connections in the brain stem. Imagine a faulty piece of electrical wiring that causes the lights to flicker on and off.

If you suffer from this, the tremor is most noticeable when you are actively keeping your body in a certain position – for example, reaching out for something – or when you are moving a part of your body. This is called an 'intention tremor' and is very different from the type that occurs in Parkinson's disease, which is most evident at rest and usually disappears with movement.

Treatment is difficult and the results are usually quite disappointing, but fortunately, a very disabling tremor is not often seen in people with MS.

Speech problems and MS

MS has the potential to affect the control of most muscles, so it is not surprising that it can affect those muscles that control voice production. As with other symptoms of MS, problems with speech can vary, particularly in the earlier stages of the condition.

Slurred speech, or speech that is difficult to understand, is fairly common in MS. It tends to be worse if you are feeling tired or stressed, anxious or feeling otherwise unwell, and it can be hard to cope with – especially when others don't understand and jump to wild conclusions. This can lead to self-consciousness, which in turn might make you feel even more stressed and worked up. Without support and advice, a vicious circle can easily develop with increased levels of frustration.

What can help?

By talking to the MS nurse or neurologist, a referral can be made to a speech therapist. They will assess the extent of the problem and provide appropriate advice, support and exercises which can improve speech problems considerably.

Case study

'I've had MS for almost 20 years now. My first symptom was weakness in my right leg which stopped me from getting about or driving for while, but it got better gradually over a few weeks.

'After that I had no obvious symptoms for about eight years but then within the space of a few years I experienced double vision, vertigo and muscle spasms. When I am tired or run down, my vision sometimes gets worse and I can get stabbing pains behind my right eye, but I know it will pass and try to take it easy.

'I find swimming and Pilates really help to keep muscle spasms at bay. If I am worried, I get in touch with my MS nurse for advice.' AB.

Summing Up

- Most people diagnosed with MS will never need to use a wheelchair on a regular basis.

- Mobility issues are not only caused by weakness or stiffness in the legs, but can also be due to problems with balance, co-ordination, dizziness or eyesight.

- Cramps, muscle stiffness and weakness are caused following inflammatory damage to the nerves in the spinal cord. They can require early support from a multidisciplinary team of health professionals, including input from a physiotherapist.

- Problems with balance, co-ordination and eyesight can be caused as a result of inflammatory damage in the brainstem and normally get better over weeks or months.

- Tremor in MS is rarely disabling and usually confined to the arms. It is caused by inflammatory damage to part of the brain called the cerebellum, or its connections to the brain.

- Speech problems in MS are caused by damage to nerves controlling voice production. Speech therapists can provide advice, support and exercises to help.

7

The Less 'Visible' Side of MS

J ust as we cannot always tell what someone is thinking, it is by no means easy to tell how or when a person's MS symptoms are affecting them.

Many people with MS experience other less visible symptoms which can be just as challenging as those mentioned in the previous chapter. However, due to lack of awareness amongst the wider population, support and understanding are sometimes in short supply.

These symptoms can include pain and altered sensations, swallowing difficulties, bladder and bowel problems and problems with sexual function.

Pain and sensations

Just as we cannot always tell what someone is thinking, it is by no means easy to tell how or when a person's MS symptoms are affecting them.

For many years, pain was not even recognised as a symptom of MS, but it is now understood that chronic pain is experienced by about 50% of people with MS. There are two different types:

Neuropathic pain

This is caused directly by inflammatory damage to the nerves and is associated with stabbing pains, extreme skin sensitivity and burning sensations. The two most common types of nerve pain experienced in MS are:

- Dysaesthesia – this is the most common form of nerve pain in MS and is an abnormal burning, pricking or stabbing sensation usually affecting the lower limbs.

- Allodynia – abnormally painful hot and cold sensations occurring when the nerves that normally send messages to the brain when the skin is wet, cold or hot suddenly start to send messages all at the same time for no apparent reason.

- Neuralgia – dagger-like pains caused by the damaged nerves misfiring for no apparent reason, even in a part of the body that is usually numb.

- Trigeminal neuralgia – electric-shock like or sharp stabbing pains experienced usually around the cheek or jaw area which can occur without any particular trigger.

Drugs for neuropathic pain

Standard pain-killers do not work for nerve pain and there are few licensed drugs in the UK for its treatment. Most of these are actually anti-epilepsy drugs which work by raising the threshold at which the nerves activate to carry messages, thereby reducing irritability. These include:

- Gabapentin (Neurontin).

- Pregabalin (Lyrica).

- Carbamazepine (Tegretol).

- Phenytoin (Epanutin).

Certain types of drugs that are actually antidepressants can sometimes be used to treat nerve pain. These include:

- Amitriptyline.

- Nortriptyline.

All the above drugs are used strictly as prescribed by your doctor and are usually started at a very low dose in order to avoid side effects such as drowsiness.

Drug treatments for nerve pain usually take the edge off the pain rather than stopping it completely, but even a small reduction in pain severity can make a big difference to your quality of life.

Some people find complementary or alternative therapies such as acupuncture or transcutaneous nerve stimulation (TENS) helps to alleviate nerve pain. In some areas, this is available through the NHS. Some neurology clinics have access to a clinical nurse specialist with expertise in pain management who can advise on this.

Regular exercise, such as swimming, is one of the best ways of managing this type of pain at an early stage. Prevention is better than cure.

Musculoskeletal pain

This is not caused directly by MS but can develop through altered posture and positioning, leading to damaged tendons, ligaments, muscles or bones.

Regular exercise, such as swimming, is one of the best ways of managing this type of pain at an early stage. Prevention is better than cure. Input from a physiotherapist (if possible, a neuro-physiotherapist) may also be helpful, as they can carry out an assessment of your posture and walking patterns and recommend a programme of exercises which can usually be continued at home. It is important if you have this type of pain to try to reserve time and energy to carry out these exercises in order to maximise benefits.

If the above measures are not enough, any of the following drug treatments may also be considered by your doctor:

- Baclofen (Lioresal).

- Dantrolene (Dantrium).

- Tizanidine (Zanaflex).

Case study

SM was diagnosed in 2004 when she was 34 years old.

'My MS manifests itself through pain and fatigue. The pain lives with me constantly. I take several neurological pain-killers and have acupuncture every other month on the area that hurts the most at that time.

'When I wake up in the morning my feet hurt even before I get out of bed and then other parts of my body take it in turns to hurt for seconds, minutes, hours or even days. I never know which part of my body is going to hurt next.

'In the first years after my diagnosis, I spent a lot of time mourning what I could no longer do and what I "used to love doing" like walking and canoeing with my family or gardening. Then my MS nurse referred me to the pain clinic. A nurse who specialised in MS pain was amazing and changed the way I thought and felt about my pain. I began concentrating on the things I "could" do and how I could adapt things so that I could still do things that I enjoyed but in a slightly different way.

'Living with pain caused by MS does not mean the end of all you enjoy in life. I've certainly done the most amazing things despite mine.' SM.

Swallowing difficulties

Over half of people with MS are likely to experience problems with eating and swallowing. Liquids tend to cause more problems than solids because they pass through the mouth faster, before the slower moving muscles have a chance to co-ordinate swallowing. This can cause coughing and choking as liquids may run into the airway to the lungs.

Some of the following suggestions may help:

- Adapt meal times to avoid eating when tired. Most MS symptoms are at their worst when you are feeling tired, unwell or emotional.

- Identify triggers which make the problem worse – if drinks are causing a difficulty, it can help to try drinks with added texture such as smoothies, pulped orange juice or milkshakes.

- Experiment with different types of drinks containers in order to find one that reduces problems.

- Sitting upright with your chin tucked when eating and drinking ensures the oesophagus is nicely aligned.

- Clearing each mouthful of food or drink from your mouth and throat before taking another reduces the likelihood of problems with swallowing.

Advice should always be sought from a healthcare professional. You may even be referred to a speech and language therapist who is trained to deal with swallowing problems as well as those specifically relating to speech.

The solution to your swallowing problems may be unexpected – singing lessons can help relieve the symptoms of choking!

Bladder and bowel problems

Bladder and bowel difficulties are very common in MS and also one of the most difficult problems to talk about. This is one area of MS where many people may attempt to suffer on in silence, but there is a great deal that can be done to help, so it is therefore important to discuss concerns with your MS nurse, neurologist or GP as soon as difficulties arise.

Bladder

If you are experiencing bladder problems, you might be referred to a specialist nurse (a continence advisor) who will assess your difficulties and discuss appropriate treatment options.

Bladder problems occur in MS as a result of damage to nerves controlling the relevant muscles, and can include:

- Needing to pass urine more often than usual (urinary frequency).
- A feeling of needing to pass water urgently (urinary urgency).
- Being unable to pass urine despite feeling the urge (urinary hesitancy).
- Passing water involuntarily, leading to accidents (urinary incontinence).

A continence advisor may carry out a bladder scan to assess the amount of urine in your bladder before and after you have passed urine. This will enable the advisor to provide the most appropriate treatment and avoid future risk of urine infections, which can cause a temporary worsening of MS symptoms if left untreated.

It is important to try and drink at least 1.5 litres of fluid each day, including drinks, soup, sauces and milk on cereal in order to stay hydrated and flush out bugs which may otherwise cause an infection.

Bowels

People with MS often have problems with their bowels. Constipation is one of the most common symptoms, occurring as a result of weakness or spasm in the muscles of the gut. Things that can help include:

- Drinking plenty of fluids – at least 1.5 litres each day.
- Eating a diet rich in fruit, vegetables and other fibre.
- Staying as active as possible – include exercises to help with posture.
- Getting into a routine of emptying your bowels each day.

If bowel problems are experienced, it is important to discuss them with a health professional before trying alternatives such as laxatives.

Sexual function

It is believed that up to 50% of people with MS will experience sexual problems at some stage in their condition, some being a direct result of MS and others having a more indirect cause. However, not all sexual problems are linked to MS – approximately 40% of the general public will have sexual problems at some time in their life.

Problems may include, or be made worse, by the following:

- Lack of libido (sex drive).
- Difficulty achieving or maintaining an erection.
- Fatigue.
- Muscle cramps (spasticity).
- Bladder problems.
- Low mood.

It is important to talk through any problems you are having and the way you are feeling with your partner and remain open and honest with each other. It may also be worth seeking advice from a healthcare professional such as your MS nurse about this sensitive issue. They can often help to put things in perspective, or arrange a referral for specialist help if needed.

There are a number of different approaches which can be helpful in resolving sexual functioning:

- Problems caused directly by MS such as bladder problems, muscle spasms and fatigue can be treated in order to ease difficulties.
- Other direct problems such as erectile dysfunction (caused by damage to the nerve connections between the brain, spinal cord and penis) can be treated by drugs such as Viagra. These can be prescribed by your GP if it is felt to be appropriate.
- There are a number of specialist clinics where couples can be shown techniques such as 'body mapping'. This can help with arousal where sensation is affected by MS.
- Counselling can be helpful for some couples in dealing with emotional concerns such as low self-esteem, changes in role and loss of desire.

There are many useful booklets about sexual function and MS available from both the MS Trust and MS Society – full contact details can be found in the help list.

Summing Up

- Nerve pain in MS is caused by inflammatory damage to nerves and is associated with stabbing pains, extreme skin sensitivity and altered sensations.

- Standard pain-killers do not work for nerve pain, but drugs normally used to treat epilepsy are sometimes prescribed if it is felt they will be beneficial.

- Musculoskeletal pain can develop through altered posture and positioning, leading to damaged tendons, ligaments, muscles or bones.

- Swallowing difficulties are likely to be experienced by more than half of people with MS, particularly with liquids rather than solids.

- Bladder problems can occur in MS as a result of inflammatory damage to nerves controlling the relevant muscles. Help can be obtained from a continence advisor.

- Difficulties with sexual function are more likely to occur in people with MS than in the wider population. It is important to talk through problems and seek advice from a health professional.

8

The 'Hidden' Side to MS

The same process of inflammatory nerve damage that causes mobility problems may also affect the channels through which energy, thoughts and emotions pass around the body.

Hidden symptoms such as fatigue, cognition and mood are often overlooked when compared to more obvious physical difficulties, but learning to recognise and understand them is a key part of living well with MS.

Without the right help at the right time, these hidden symptoms can stunt your future well before the physical condition can.

Fatigue

What is fatigue?

Many people find it a relief to discover that fatigue is a recognised symptom of MS but find this "invisible" symptom hard to describe.

Fatigue is an unpredictable, debilitating form of tiredness experienced at some time by the majority of people with MS. It is more than the tiredness felt after a hard day at work. Many people find it a relief to discover that it is a recognised effect of MS.

In the same way that damaged electrical wiring can cause a light to flicker on and off, damaged nerves can affect how energy is passed around the body.

The contrast between what someone can achieve when energy gets through to when it doesn't can be one of the most frustrating things about MS – and also one of the most confusing for other people to understand.

What fatigue is not!

Fatigue is not laziness or a convenient excuse for special treatment. Laziness, on the other hand, is a mental attitude linked to inertia (disinterest), apathy (lack of concern) and lack of voluntary effort that can be overcome with willpower.

Try not to compare your existing energy levels with what they used to be, or to those of other people around you. It can take time, but if you can learn to measure your life by your own individual accomplishments, rather than other people's, it will help you to manage your MS.

What causes fatigue in MS?

Research into the link between MS and fatigue is ongoing, but it is thought that a combination of the following factors may contribute:

- Nerves that have lost their myelin insulation might still be able to function normally up to a point, but become exhausted if they have to work too hard.

- There is a possibility that the immune system itself might release chemicals that cause a feeling of fatigue.

- Because of damage to the nerve pathways, people with MS may have to use more parts of their brain to achieve the same result as someone who does not have MS.

- Other MS symptoms like muscle weakness, stiffness, pain, tremor and depression may lead to feelings of fatigue if not treated and managed.

- Living with MS can have knock-on effects resulting in lack of or disturbed sleep, lower energy levels, anxiety and low mood. These can all cause feelings of fatigue.

Can fatigue be treated?

If fatigue is affecting your home or work life, it is important to speak to your MS nurse or doctor. To help them assess whether your fatigue is caused directly by your MS, you may be shown how to complete a fatigue diary for a period of time. This might include some of the following information:

- The time of day when your fatigue is at its worst.

- Any particular tasks at work or at home that bring on fatigue.

- Fatigue levels after exercise.

- Medications you are taking – what they are for and when you take them.

- Sleep problems – any particular cause you can think of or pattern that has developed.

- The possibility of an infection which may need to be ruled out.

- Feelings of anxiety, low mood and depression.

- Any other health problems, such as shortness of breath.

Most people with MS seem to have a strong work ethic and a desire to achieve their goals.

Having identified and tackled fatigue caused either by other MS symptoms, living with the condition or by factors unrelated to MS, if you are still experiencing fatigue then this might be linked directly to the effects of MS on the central nervous system.

Health professionals working within the multidisciplinary neurology team can provide advice on several strategies which can help to manage fatigue, including:

- The importance of rest and how to build it in to your lifestyle.
- Prioritising tasks in order to make the most of energy reserves.
- Asking for help – the right sort at the right times.
- Planning your time more effectively.
- Organising your living and work spaces.
- Maintaining good posture when standing and sitting.
- Sensible exercise and healthy eating.

Cognition is used to describe our ability to do a wide range of tasks such as communicate, recognise things, remember, learn and plan.

Are there any drugs for fatigue?

Fatigue is a difficult symptom to manage and at present there is no reliably effective medication that can help.

Certain drugs licensed for other conditions are sometimes prescribed:

- Ammantadine (Symmetrel or Lysovir) appears to benefit only a minority of people with MS and side effects can include insomnia and vivid dreams.
- Modafinil (Provigil) has not proven to be very effective in trials with MS, although some who have taken it say they benefited.
- Prokarin (sometimes spelt Procarin) is a skin patch containing caffeine and histamine. It is not available on prescription as trials so far have not proven benefits for treating MS fatigue.

Memory and thought processing

Amongst the many new terms you will probably come across at some point is the word 'cognition'. It is used to describe our ability to do a wide range of tasks such as communicate, recognise things, remember, learn and plan.

Cognition is another invisible symptom of MS that is often much overlooked, but recent research has shown that a wide range of cognitive problems might be experienced by up to 65% of people with MS. Most people will only experience mild to moderate problems on a temporary basis, but these can nevertheless have an impact on your ability to work, socialise and enjoy leisure time.

What causes cognitive changes in MS?

The brain is a complex network of nerves that are linked, communicating with each other and with parts of the body. In MS, patches of inflammatory nerve damage can disrupt and slow down these communications, causing problems with memory and thinking.

Cognitive problems in MS can lead to difficulties with:

- Focusing, maintaining and shifting one's attention.
- Learning, remembering and recalling information.
- Understanding and using language appropriately and effectively.
- Performing maths calculations.
- Executive functioning – planning, sorting and multi-tasking.

Unfortunately, society at large sometimes stigmatises people who have problems in these areas, thinking of them as stupid, lazy or even rude. It is important that people around you are made aware that cognitive problems such as these are due to your MS.

There aren't any drug treatments at present to help with cognitive problems, but a clinical psychologist, possibly from within your multidisciplinary healthcare team, can provide advice.

Many people with MS have learned useful 'compensatory strategies', such as applying themselves to one task at a time rather than constantly flitting from one thing to another. Many more tips like this can be found on the new MS Trust website (www.stayingsmart.org.uk) where people can share useful information and build confidence in managing cognitive difficulties in MS.

Emotions

Just as everyone's experience of MS is different, so we all have different personalities, coping styles and strengths. Nobody can control every emotion and remain positive and happy all the time, but there are strategies that can be used to prepare for and manage some of the emotional effects of MS.

Fear and anxiety

About a third of people with MS are affected by anxiety. These are understandable emotions to experience when faced with the diagnosis of an unpredictable condition. It is important to remember not to struggle on alone, as there are many strategies that can help to manage these emotions, including:

- Setting a worry time each day – five minutes each morning and evening.
- Sharing fear – telling others can help to keep things in perspective.
- Writing a list of coping strategies and keeping it where you can see it.
- Recognising how your thoughts can affect your feelings and emotions.
- Learning new thinking patterns by finding positive answers to negative thoughts.

If fear and anxiety begin to feel overwhelming, it is important to seek help from your GP, MS nurse or other health or social care professional. Some people find it helpful to talk to a clinical psychologist who understands MS and the emotions it can cause.

Studies have not as yet proven a definite link between stress and MS, but it is widely recognised that stress affects the body's ability to fight disease.

Stress

Stress is a normal part of everyday life for everyone, but in addition to facing normal stresses, people with MS have to deal with the unpredictability and pressures the condition itself causes. This can include the ability to work, thought processing, friendships and relationships, housework and parenting.

Studies have not as yet proven a definite link between stress and MS, but it is widely recognised that stress affects the body's ability to fight disease. Learning to recognise the connection between stress and worsening of symptoms can help you to feel more in control of your MS.

It is impossible to eliminate stress totally from your life but there are many stress management techniques you can employ to help manage it and take back control. These include:

- Learning to recognise what you can control and what you can't control.
- Seeking support from someone you trust.
- Setting realistic goals and planning ahead.
- Challenging your negative thinking styles.

- Keeping a stress diary for two months.
- Becoming more aware of how different roles and relationships affect you.
- Considering complementary therapies.
- Carrying out sensible exercise.
- Finding ordinary, everyday activities that are enjoyable to you.
- Teaching yourself relaxation and calm breathing techniques.

For more information see Stress – The Essential Guide (Need2Know).

Mood swings

People with MS do seem to have mood swings more often than other people. As with depression, it might be that mood swings happen because of a person's reaction to having MS, but they can also be a direct result of nerve damage on the front parts of the brain which control mood.

The same processes can also cause some people to laugh or cry uncontrollably, but it is rare for this to be a severe or persistent problem.

Your MS nurse or GP may suggest counselling, cognitive behavioural therapy or antidepressant medication if your mood swings are becoming difficult to manage.

Depression

Of the general population, 10% will have a major depressive episode during their lifetime. If you have MS, the odds are much higher, with up to 50% experiencing a major depressive episode in their lifetime (Minden, 1999). Depression is often unrecognised by both people with MS and healthcare professionals, yet once addressed can usually be successfully treated.

What is depression?

According to the MS Society, depression is defined as a disorder characterised by a 'persistently low mood most of the time, lasting for a few weeks or more'. It can cause distress and affect social and work abilities, with sadness and emptiness accompanying low mood.

It can be difficult to diagnose depression in MS because some of the MS symptoms such as fatigue, sleeplessness or loss of libido can imitate symptoms of depression.

Your doctor will make an assessment based on how long you have experienced at least half of the following symptoms:

- Feelings of hopelessness, sadness or despair.
- Loss of pleasure or interest in most daily activities.
- Significant weight loss or gain; or an increase or decrease in appetite.
- Persistent sleep problems, either insomnia or excessive sleep.
- Ongoing fatigue and loss of energy.
- Feelings of personal worthlessness.
- Inappropriate and excessive guilt.
- Inability to concentrate or make decisions.
- Observable restlessness or slowed movement.
- Recurrent thoughts of death, violence or suicide.

It is important to seek help immediately from your GP if you feel you might have depression.

What causes depression in MS?

Living with an unpredictable, long-term condition can understandably make a person depressed, but in MS there are certain additional factors that might also be responsible for periods of depression:

- Diagnosis itself can understandably cause periods of sadness.
- Changes in physical or cognitive abilities.
- Relapses and the increased unpredictability they can bring.
- MS damage to the emotional centres of the brain.
- Side effects of medication.

Treatments for depression

Research indicates that the best way to treat depression is to use a combination of medication and therapy, including:

- Addressing the root causes and making appropriate changes in social support.
- Antidepressant medication – this can take several weeks to start working.
- Individual or family counselling.
- Self-help strategies, including sensible exercise and developing new skills.

For more information see Depression – The Essential Guide (Need2Know).

Summing Up

- Hidden symptoms such as fatigue, cognition and mood are often overlooked compared to the more physically challenging symptoms.

- Learning to recognise and understand these hidden symptoms is a key part of living well with MS and is as important as managing the more physical symptoms.

- Fatigue is an unpredictable, overwhelming form of tiredness experienced at some time by the majority of people with MS and recognised as a symptom of the condition.

- Health professionals working within the multidisciplinary neurology team will be able to provide advice and strategies to manage the impact of fatigue.

- Fear, anxiety, stress, depression or mood swings can occur indirectly or directly as a result of MS. They can often be treated successfully through either drug treatment or talking therapies.

- Memory and thought processing problems are experienced by up to 65% of people with MS, with most only experiencing mild to moderate problems, for which compensatory strategies can be helpful.

9

Relapses

n the previous three chapters we looked at the wide range of symptoms that can be experienced in MS and treatments used. In this chapter we will be explaining the relationship between symptoms and relapses, how relapses are managed and when a relapse may not be a 'true' relapse.

In order to appreciate the complexity of managing relapses in MS, we will first recap some important facts.

A reminder of some important facts...

People can fully recover from relapses not only when there is myelin damage, but even if nerve fibres themselves are damaged.

- MS is a condition of the central nervous system and can therefore affect any of the body's actions and activities; including movement, balance, thought processes and emotions.

- Location, severity and duration of symptoms are unpredictable and will vary from person to person.

- Symptoms are caused by damage from inflammatory cells attacking the nerve fibres in the brain and spinal cord. This attack results in fluid collecting around the nerve fibre, compressing the nerve and preventing messages getting through to parts of the body.

- When the fluid disappears and no longer compresses the nerve fibres, then there is remission. Inflammation can damage the myelin sheath around the nerve fibres, the nerve fibres themselves or even the nerves cells.

Looking again at these facts can help us to see that when making decisions about treatments and drugs, health professionals are faced with a significant number of variable factors – MS is not a 'one size fits all' condition.

In order to make appropriate decisions about treatment, neurologists and MS nurses will use their knowledge and experience, along with any test results, your medical history and what you tell them about your symptoms.

What is a relapse?

A relapse can also be referred to as an attack, a bout, an episode or an exacerbation of MS. It is usually defined as the occurrence of new symptoms or the recurrence of old symptoms that last more than 24 hours and occur more than a month after a previous episode.

Although studies have not yet shown any specific, convincing trigger factors in MS, relapses can often follow infections, particularly urinary tract and respiratory infections. Therefore, if you have MS, it's important to obtain early treatment for bacterial infections.

What happens during a relapse?

During a relapse, symptoms will typically:

- Develop gradually over a short period of time – hours or days.
- Stabilise over a number of weeks.
- Vary from mild to severe.
- Improve over weeks or months.
- Begin to settle down or disappear (this is known as remission).

In the early stages of relapsing remitting MS, recovery from relapses is complete or substantial more than 80% of the time. As time goes by, and if further relapses occur, you may experience further symptoms even during remission due to incomplete recovery from relapses.

Remissions can last any length of time – even years. It is not possible to predict the extent of recovery from a relapse or whether a person may experience a temporary recurrence or worsening of symptoms during periods of remission.

If your condition starts to deteriorate slowly between relapses, this indicates that a critical number of axons (nerve fibres) may have been damaged or destroyed in a particular part of the central nervous system.

If there has been clear evidence of sustained deterioration for at least six months, which is completely independent of the effect of relapses, it can be said that a person has moved from relapsing remitting MS to secondary progressive.

Treatment options

Relapses with milder symptoms

If the symptoms are mild, have been present for only a day or two and relate to alteration or loss of sensation, your MS nurse or doctor may suggest the following, simple, short-term measures:

- Resting.
- Eating regularly.
- Getting plenty of sleep.

If your symptoms continue to worsen and are affecting your day-to-day life, you should contact your health professionals again so that they can reassess your situation.

Severe relapses

Steroids

There is often much confusion amongst MS patients about the use of steroids in the treatment of relapses. If MS symptoms are causing particular distress and/ or taking a long time to disappear, you might find it confusing that doctors don't use the same approach as last time. You may even wonder if drugs are being withheld to save money. This is not the case!

Here are some facts about steroids which should help to clarify things:

- Steroids work by dampening down inflammation, much as a steroid cream might be used for treating an inflammatory skin condition such as eczema. This can help to speed up recovery from the relapse, but there is no evidence that they make any difference to the long-term course of the condition.

- Steroids can only work in this way if inflammation truly exists. Most people can understand that steroid skin cream would not be prescribed for an old scar which may have healed years before. The principle is the same, but it is harder to understand because MS inflammation is happening inside the body and cannot be seen.

- Steroids are probably most effective when used early in the course of a relapse.

- Steroids can also have many side effects. In the short term, they can cause a metallic taste in the mouth, flushing to the face and body, mood swings, dyspepsia (indigestion and reflux) and sleep deprivation.

- Frequent and prolonged use of steroids can increase the risk of bone thinning (osteoporosis), bone death (avascular necrosis), fractures, muscle wasting, stomach ulcers and infections.

Doctors will normally only prescribe steroids if a patient is experiencing significant new symptoms of a true relapse, with symptoms so disabling as to significantly interfere with a person's day-to-day life, i.e. unable to walk, go to work or in distressing pain.

Many doctors recommend no more than two courses of high dose steroids in any 12 month period, except in very unusual circumstances.

How are steroids given?

There are many treatment regimes around the UK, but the most common steroid used is methylprednisolone which can be given in two different ways:

- In tablet form – 500mg per day for five days.
- By intravenous drip into a vein – this can require hospital admission.

Side effects are common and include poor sleep, mental agitation, euphoria and feeling flushed. Some people find they have fewer side effects with one form than with the other, and occasionally people can find that the side effects of steroids feel worse than the MS symptoms they were experiencing.

It is important that you discuss any concerns with your doctor or MS nurse who will decide on the best treatment regime for you as an individual.

Steroids can only work if inflammation truly exists.

'Pseudo-relapses'

This is a term used to describe a worsening of symptoms or the return of old symptoms, but where new inflammation is not the cause.

Steroids will be of no benefit with a pseudo-relapse as inflammation is not the cause of symptoms and the risk of side effects would be experienced unnecessarily.

For a person living with MS, pseudo-relapses can be confusing and frightening if they do not understand what is happening but are simply told that steroids will not help.

There are no hard and fast rules to differentiate a true relapse from a pseudo-relapse, but the characteristics of a pseudo-relapse can include:

- A recurrence of old symptoms.
- A worsening of long-standing symptoms.

- Symptoms only lasting a few hours or coming and going on a day-to-day basis.

- A recent infection or particularly stressful time.

Exercise and hot temperatures may also cause a brief re-emergence of old symptoms previously experienced during a relapse. For example, a person may experience blurred vision temporarily in one eye which was previously affected by optic neuritis (see p.52). This is known as 'Uthoff's' phenomenon.

Summing Up

- MS is not a 'one size fits all' condition. There are a significant number of variable factors that health professionals have to take into account when prescribing treatment for relapses.

- A relapse can also be referred to as an attack, a bout, an episode or an exacerbation of symptoms lasting more than 24 hours.

- Relapses can often follow infections, so it is important for you to obtain early treatment for bacterial infections.

- Steroids can have many side effects and are only effective in speeding up recovery times in true relapses where inflammation is present.

- Steroids are normally given in tablet form or by intravenous drip.

- Pseudo-relapses are a worsening of symptoms or the return of old symptoms that come and go. Symptoms are not caused by inflammation but are the result of other factors such as infection, stress or heat.

- Steroids will be of no benefit with a pseudo-relapse.

10

Can MS be Stopped from Getting Worse?

Scientists have yet to find a cure for MS or develop treatments that can regenerate damaged nerve cells. But our understanding of the best ways of managing the condition is improving all the time and several potential new drug therapies are currently in development.

We have already looked at treatments for symptoms and relapses. In this chapter, we are going to look at the 'third strand' of treatment in MS: disease modifying drugs (DMDs). Unlike the drugs that are used to treat symptoms and relapses, DMDs affect the long-term course of MS.

It is important to emphasise that although the information contained here may help you to understand more about these drugs, it is not a substitute for clinical advice. When it comes to making decisions about treatments, the partnership between you and your health professionals is vital.

Our understanding of the best ways of managing the condition is improving all the time and several potential new drug therapies are currently in development.

Disease modifying drugs

Who is eligible for DMDs?

Results from clinical trials support the use of DMDs in:

- People with relapsing remitting MS who have had two or more relapses in two years and can walk 100-200m.

- People with progressive relapsing MS who have had two or more relapses in two years and can still walk 10m.

How do DMDs work?

Unlike steroids which dampen down inflammation once a relapse has already begun, DMDs work by reducing the inflammatory processes that can cause relapses to happen in the first place.

For a non-medical person, this can sometimes be a hard concept to grasp because it is all taking place inside the body.

Some important facts about DMDs:

- It is important to recognise that DMDs are not a cure for MS; they can neither halt the progress or reverse the damage that has already occurred in MS.

- DMDs act in different ways. Not every person with MS will benefit from, or even respond to, the drugs in the same way.

How will I know which drug is best for me?

Before starting treatment, you will attend a number of assessments, meetings and discussions with your neurologist and also your MS nurse. You will have an opportunity to seek answers to any questions you still have about the drugs, including the practicalities of starting treatment and how it will fit in with your lifestyle.

- Blood tests will be performed before treatment commences in order to check for any problems that might affect how well you do on the drugs. You will also be asked about any pre-existing conditions or reactions to previous drugs or treatments.

- Most of the existing treatments are taken by injection and one is taken by intravenous drip. However, clinical trials currently taking place indicate that an oral treatment may be licensed for use in the very near future.

DMDs work by reducing the inflammatory processes that can cause relapses to happen in the first place.

- Although you need to give due consideration to how these drugs fit with your priorities, goals and lifestyle choices, it is important that you are also aware of the mounting evidence to suggest that the earlier treatment commences, the more effective the drugs can be.

- If you are considering treatment with the licensed DMDs referred to in this chapter, there is a web-based patient decision aid called MS Decisions (see help list). Information can also be obtained from the websites of the MS Society and the MS Trust (see help list).

Beta interferon

Beta interferon has been used in the UK and the US for over 15 years and has established a very good safety profile. There are two different types of interferon beta used in the treatment of MS (the differences between them lie in the way they are manufactured).

- Beta interferon 1a has two different brand names: Avonex and Rebif.

- Beta interferon 1b also has two different brand names: Betaferon and Extavia.

All of these drugs are licensed for use in relapsing remitting MS. Studies have shown a reduction in the rate of disease progression and a reduction in the frequency and severity of relapses of around one third.

- Betaferon, Rebif and Extavia are licensed for use in secondary progressive MS where relapses are still occurring. They have been shown to reduce the frequency and severity of relapses.
- Avonex, Betaferon and Extavia are licensed for use in CIS. They have been shown to delay progression from CIS to clinically definite MS.

How do beta interferon drugs work in MS?

In time, some people learn to view their injections as a way of taking back some control of their MS, instead of it seeming like a one-sided battle.

Interferons are proteins produced naturally by the human body. They help to fight infections and play an important role in the functioning of the immune system. There are three types of natural interferon: alpha, gamma and beta.

- Alpha interferons are used in the treatment of some types of cancers but have not proven beneficial in the treatment of MS.
- Gamma interferons are thought to stimulate MS symptoms.
- Beta interferons are thought to work by blocking the actions of the gamma interferons thereby reducing the autoimmune reaction, which alleviates symptoms.

How are beta interferon drugs given?

All the beta interferon drugs are self-administered and given by injection either under the skin or into the muscle. Depending on which drug is prescribed, this is done either three times a week, on alternate days, or once a week.

People who are anxious about injections often choose to use auto-injectors. These are available for all the self-administered drugs and work like a pen which holds a needle and syringe inside. Most types of auto-injector allow you to inject without having to see the needle going in.

Your MS nurse will show you how to prepare for the injection, how to administer it and how to deal with any side effects. In time, some people learn to view their injections as a way of taking back some control of their MS, instead of it seeming like a one-sided battle.

Side effects of beta interferon drugs

More often than not, the side effects of these drugs are mild and manageable, mainly consisting of flu like symptoms after injecting or injection site reactions (e.g. swelling or bruising).

- There are various strategies that your MS nurse may recommend in order to reduce the risk of experiencing side effects whilst on these drugs.

- If family, friends and colleagues are aware that you may need additional support and understanding while your body gets used to the medication, that will also help you to adjust.

- Other side effects from interferons can include anaemia and liver dysfunction, so regular blood tests are carried out.

What if beta interferon stops working?

Any person starting drug treatment needs to understand that while these drug treatments are a long-term commitment, they are not necessarily a lifelong commitment. While these drugs might prove effective over a long period of time, they will not necessarily maintain the same level of effectiveness.

One reason for reduced effectiveness is the development of antibodies. These are proteins produced by the immune system to fight foreign substances such as infections. In MS they can have the effect of blocking the benefits of beta interferon.

Your neurologist may perform a blood test from time to time in order to check for these neutralising antibodies. They are not experienced by the majority of patients, might even disappear again over time and are not a reason for stopping or changing drugs.

Glatiramer acetate

This drug works differently to beta interferon. It is thought to prevent the production of myelin reactive immune cells (cells responsible for the destruction of myelin) and encourages the generation of anti-inflammatory immune cells. This combined effect dampens down the inflammation occurring in the central nervous system, thereby reducing the damage to myelin and nerve fibres.

Glatiramer acetate (brand name Copaxone) has also been used in the UK and the US for over 15 years and has established a very good safety record. It is licensed for use in:

- Relapsing remitting MS, where it has been shown to reduce the frequency and severity of relapses by around one-third in this patient group.

- CIS, where early treatment has been shown to delay progression to a more active form of MS.

Glatiramer acetate can have a six month delay before benefits are seen. It is self-administered by injection under the skin every day. Common side effects are injection site reactions and indentations in the skin.

Less common side effects are post injection reactions in the form of chest tightness, breathlessness, anxiety, flushing and palpitations which all typically pass after a few minutes. It is important to speak to your MS nurse if you have concerns as there are various strategies that they can recommend in order to reduce the risk of experiencing side effects.

Natalizumab

Natalizumab (brand name Tysabri) is one of the most recent DMDs to be approved in the UK for the treatment of MS. It is given in hospital as an intravenous infusion (a needle placed in a vein, similar to a drip) once every four weeks.

Before each treatment session, blood pressure, temperature and pulse rates will be taken. A nurse or doctor will monitor the infusion, which usually takes one hour, and for one hour after the infusion to check for any signs or symptoms of allergic reactions.

Natalizumab is licensed only for the following MS groups:

- Patients experiencing increasing MS symptoms despite treatment with beta interferon.

- Patients with rapidly evolving severe relapsing remitting MS.

Studies have shown natalizumab to:

- Reduce the occurrences of relapses by around two-thirds.

- Significantly reduce the rate of disease progression.

Side effects

Natalizumab is designed to treat more active forms of MS and has a more toxic effect on the body. Side effects can include:

- Reactions to the infusions.

- Allergic reactions.

- Serious infections, including PML (progressive multifocal leukoencephalopathy), a rare brain infection that can lead to severe disability or even death.

In view of the risks associated with serious infections, particularly PML, individuals are subject to close clinical monitoring and issued with a patient alert card designed to help them identify any potentially serious side effects.

Persistent presence of neutralising antibodies can reduce effectiveness and also increase the risk of hypersensitivity reactions. If blood tests show that neutralising antibodies are persistently present then treatment is discontinued.

'Off-label' prescribing

There are certain exceptional circumstances when drugs that are not licensed for MS may be used. Such recommendations would be made on an individual patient basis, and are decided by the prescribing doctor.

Some of these drugs may be licensed for treatment of other autoimmune diseases such as rheumatoid arthritis and the skin condition psoriasis, but are occasionally used 'off-label' for treatment of MS. This means that there is insufficient data to prove how safe or effective the drug is when used for MS.

Mitoxantrone is a chemotherapy drug that is used 'off-label' at some of the larger neurology centres in the UK for severe, rapidly progressing or unresponsive cases of MS. It can have many severe side effects so has to be monitored very carefully.

Case study

'I have been on beta interferon 1b since 1997. Prior to receiving the treatment I was having two or three major relapses per year, causing me to be off sick from work for 6-8 weeks on each occasion. After commencing injections I was able to continue at work for another eight years until I retired. I now have only occasional minor relapses lasting a couple of weeks at most.

'I have only had a few minor problems with self-injecting from the outset. I have always used an "auto-inject", preferring not to see the needle go in! Apart from the usual raised red areas at the injection site, the worst side effect for me is a couple of hours of chill and shivering, which thankfully only occurs once in a blue moon.' JM.

Summing Up

- Our understanding of the best ways of managing MS is improving all the time and several potential new drug therapies are currently being developed and tested.

- It is important to recognise that DMDs are not a cure for MS; they can neither halt the progress or reverse the damage that has already occurred in MS.

- Beta interferons are thought to work by blocking the actions of gamma interferons, thereby reducing the autoimmune reaction that results in inflammation and destruction of myelin.

- Benefits from DMDs range from reduced frequency and severity of relapses to delayed disease progression, depending on which drug is prescribed and which type of MS it is licensed for.

- Other drugs used in MS might include 'off label' treatments where a licence for use in MS is not held.

11

Research

Through ongoing research, we are learning more all the time about how the central nervous system works and what causes some people to be more susceptible to the development of MS.

A lot of high quality research is taking place along with many clinical trials which will lead to improved treatments in the future.

The main challenges faced by scientists

- The first is to find out what causes an attack of MS and to try to reduce the chances of it happening, thereby preventing damage to the nerves.

- The second is to try and reverse the damage already caused by previous MS attacks.

Most of the existing MS treatments have so far only been proven to reduce the frequency and number of attacks experienced by a person. They have not been shown to be effective in repairing damage to nerves which has already taken place.

The media...

MS is a high profile condition and any new research findings may be considered newsworthy and published in newspapers or broadcast on radio and television. Barely a week goes by without claims of new discoveries and breakthroughs in MS being reported in the news media.

There is no denying that the media has been a great help in raising awareness of MS, as well as raising funds for research and enabling people within the world wide MS community to link up, exchange and support each other.

However, it is important to remember that the way the media presents news can sometimes be misleading and without any factual evidence to back it up.

Although good journalists usually indicate whether research has been published and mention the name of the scientific journal it has appeared in, most of the time there is not space or interest in full references to back up these stories of cures for MS.

Most people with MS will have been passed newspaper cuttings by well-meaning friends and family with headlines such as 'Doctor discovers MS cure' followed by a short 100 words usually including the words 'according to' and 'claims'. It

> A lot of high quality research is taking place along with many clinical trials which will lead to improved treatments in the future.

is only natural for people to interpret these claims as a sign of hope, but without facts and robust evidence to back them up, it can often mean disappointment and frustration.

Types of research

At the moment there are six types of research on MS taking place.

Laboratory-based research

This can involve working with blood and tissue samples from people with MS to try and find out how and why the disease affects the central nervous system. It can provide information leading to treatments that might alter the course of the illness by protecting nerve cells from injury and death. It can also tell us about the possible genetic differences between people with and without MS.

Genetics

There has been much progress in recent years in this area of research. Genetic factors account for about one third of a person's risk of developing MS and evidence so far suggests there are at least five genes involved in determining this risk, but not necessarily the same five genes in each person.

One group of genes in particular has consistently shown an association with an increased risk of getting MS, though it is also a very common gene within the wider population. Even if people were tested and found to have this variant, they would statistically be much more likely never to develop MS, so testing for it is not generally felt to be useful.

It becomes clear that genetic research in MS presents many complex challenges, with environmental factors and luck also playing a major role. Even if we could screen a person's individual DNA, and knew all of the genes that play a role in MS and how they applied to that person, we would still only be able to give them an age-adjusted estimated risk of having or developing MS.

Epidemiological research

This looks at why MS is more common in one part of the world than another and what factors might explain these differences. For example, studies by Compston and colleagues have shown that MS seems to be more common in populations living further away from the equator. Even in the UK, MS is more common in the north, especially in Scotland where MS affects one person in every 500.

'Case-control' studies

These are studies that investigate the backgrounds of individual people in order to identify factors that may contribute to the development of MS. As it is done retrospectively, it relies on people's memories and therefore may not be a reliable source of information.

It is well recognised that people with MS can improve on a placebo even though it does not contain any active ingredients. This is known as "the placebo effect".

Applied research

This looks at interventions that might reduce the impact of symptoms or help people to manage their symptoms better. For example, speech therapy has been found to benefit patients who have experienced problems with swallowing.

Clinical research

This focuses on the 'natural development' of MS, the symptoms and signs that develop in people over time and how these may affect their ability to function in everyday life. Through clinical trials it can also examine the effectiveness and safety of potential new therapies for MS.

Clinical trials

In order to be given a licence for use in a condition, every new drug has to go through rigorous testing of its effectiveness and safety. This is done by a series of clinical trails, often over many years. A potential new medicine may be rejected at any point on the development process on safety, effectiveness or quality grounds and on average will take 10-15 years to get from the test tube to the medicine cabinet.

Clinical trials are designed to find out whether there is a difference between the effect of a treatment with a new drug and the effect of treatment with a 'dummy drug' (placebo). It is well recognised that people with MS can improve on a placebo even though it does not contain any active ingredients. This is known as 'the placebo effect'.

Any MS patient considering taking part in such a trial will need to consider the risks and implications involved. They will have to meet the relevant eligibility criteria defined by the trial investigators and will also need a referral from their neurologist or MS nurse.

According to the Clinical Trials Registry, in January 2010 there were over 500 different studies looking into some aspect or treatment of MS by organisations all around the world. Some of the more notable drugs being studied for their safety and effectiveness in relapsing remitting MS are:

- Alemtuzumab (Campath).
- BG-12.
- Cladribine (Leustat).
- Daclizumab (Zenapax).
- Fingolimod.
- Laquinimod.
- Neurovax.
- Rituximab (Rituxan).
- Teriflunomide.
- Tovaxin.

Several of the above will be prescribed in tablet form, eliminating the need for injections. Drug development for MS is fast moving and fast changing. Your consultant or MS nurse will be able to provide you with advice and information about clinical trials currently recruiting people. Further information can also be found by searching the Clinical Trials Registry online or visit the research pages of the MS Trust (see help list).

Potential treatments for symptoms

There are many other studies taking place to try and find treatments which can ease symptoms in MS, too many to mention in this book. The latest information can be found on the two websites referred to above.

Low dose naltrexone

One treatment that has been much talked about in the media recently is low dose naltrexone (LDN), a drug which has historically been used in high doses to treat addiction to codeine, morphine, heroine and alcohol. Studies have indicated that when used in significantly lower doses, naltrexone can have a beneficial impact on pain, mood, hormones and appetite as well as having an anti-inflammatory effect.

Although LDN has been used for a number of different conditions and symptoms including bladder dysfunction, fatigue and spasticity, the controlled trials evidence in MS is sparse and requires replication in much larger studies before any conclusions about its benefits can be reached.

Drug development for MS is fast moving and fast changing.

Cannabis-based medicines

Cannabis-based medicines have shown some promise when formally studied in clinical trials and one cannabis-based medicine (Sativex) has even received a preliminary licence for use with MS in Canada. Nevertheless, the results of this type of medicine in terms of the benefits for symptoms of MS have been conflicting and inconsistent and the UK drug licensing body has not yet granted a licence for any of the treatments developed so far.

Stem cell therapy

Stem cell therapy has huge potential in the treatment of MS. Stem cells are capable of renewing themselves and changing into other cells including those that make myelin. This brings the hope that one day stem cell therapy might renew damaged myelin, or even repair the malfunctioning immune system that causes inflammation in the brain and spinal cord.

Although stem cell therapy has great potential, there are a number of problems that must be overcome – including the risk of cancer and infections – before it can be shown to be both effective and safe.

Despite these risks, commercial companies are offering expensive stem cell therapy directly to people with MS, without properly assessing them neurologically either before or after treatment and against the advice of neurologists.

Chronic cerebrospinal venous insufficiency

Chronic cerebrospinal venous insufficiency (CCSVI) is a syndrome characterised by poor removal of oxygen-depleted blood from the central nervous system. This is thought to be caused by a constriction of blood vessels in the brain and neck. Some researchers have theorised that it may lead to a build-up of iron in the brain which may have a negative effect on nerve growth, leading to MS symptoms.

Trials have begun using a surgical treatment called 'balloon dilation' to improve drainage from the brain and although the results are interesting, there is not as yet enough evidence demonstrating the safety or effectiveness of this treatment in MS.

In 2009, the MS Society was funding around 80 vital MS research projects in the UK.

Summing Up

- Through ongoing research, our understanding of MS, how the central nervous system works and what causes some people to be more susceptible to the development of MS is improving all the time.

- It is important to remember that the way the media presents news can sometimes be misleading and without any factual evidence to back it up.

- Laboratory-based research can provide information leading to treatments that might alter the course of the illness by protecting nerve cells form injury and death, and also about the genetic differences between people with and without MS.

- Genetic factors account for about one third of a person's risk of developing MS and evidence so far suggests there are at least five genes involved in determining this risk, but not necessarily the same five genes in each person.

- In order to be given a licence for use in a condition, every new drug has to go through rigorous testing of its effectiveness and safety. This is done by a series of clinical trails, often over many years

- According to the Clinical Trials Registry, in January 2010 there were over 500 different studies looking into some aspect or treatment of MS by organisations all around the world.

12

Relationships

J ust as each person's experience of MS is different, so its impact on relationships will vary widely according to individual coping styles, hopes, expectations and circumstances. One thing that MS does not change is the essence of who you are.

Relationships are a key area in living well with MS and it is important not to feel isolated – help is out there.

Communication

MS can act as a magnifying glass, showing up both the positive and negative aspects of relationships which were already there before a diagnosis. It is important to be honest about your feelings. Learning and practising good communication skills can help to deal with current and future conflicts.

A few basic tips for better communication

One thing that MS does not change is the essence of who you are.

- Try to be a better listener than a talker.
- Accept support and help when offered.
- Turn the TV, computer or radio off – give the person trying to communicate all your attention.
- Recognise that men and women communicate in different ways.
- Remember that it is all right to have different opinions.

Relationships with partners

All relationships have hopes and plans for the future, a shared history and a shared commitment to making the relationship work. MS can cause a shift in these, as well as changing some of the familiar roles that partners have in a relationship, but with a flexible approach from both partners, the impact of these role changes can be easier to adapt to.

Practical roles

It would be fair to say that in most households some of the following practical roles tend to be done more regularly by one partner than the other:

- Cook.

- Computer wizard.

- Gardener.

- Cleaner.

- Driver.

- Accountant.

Some roles are physically demanding, and others require more concentration skills than physical effort. If possible, swapping some of these roles, or breaking them down into smaller parts, can better suit challenges imposed by MS such as fatigue, mobility issues or cognitive problems. This might take time to get used to, but playing to each of your strengths will encourage a positive outlook and a sense of working together as a team.

- Learning to let go of the housework so that you can spend more time doing things that are important to both of you can be very hard, but it is also worth doing. If finances allow, it might be worth considering employing a cleaner for a few hours each week to help with the particularly heavy tasks.

- Depending on the level of your disability, you might be entitled to the care component of Disability Living Allowance (DLA) to help with this type of support. Chapter 13 refers to financial matters.

- There may also be aids or equipment which could help you manage the housework more easily. Occupational therapists can provide information and practical advice on ways to adapt your home and make it easier to manage.

Playing to each of your strengths will encourage a positive outlook and a sense of working together as a team.

Emotional roles

Without realising it, we all develop invisible or emotional roles in a relationship as well as practical ones. For example, if you are the one with MS and were historically the stronger one emotionally, living with this condition may change the dimensions of your relationship.

This does not always have to be a change for the worse – some couples affected by MS say that they have both found hidden strengths that they didn't realise they had and have become closer as a result.

In time, with a flexible approach and the right help, it is possible to redefine some of the roles that underpin a relationship so that both sides retain their self-esteem and feel they can continue to make a valued contribution to the relationship.

Partner... or carer?

Sometimes a partner might provide intimate care, such as help with bathing or dressing. Although the term 'carer' can be a useful title when trying to access outside help and support, it is important to recognise that this caring role is only one part of any relationship. The factors that bonded you together before MS came along still remain.

If you feel your relationship is suffering as a result of your MS, talk to your MS nurse, GP or other health professional.

There are several organisations that exist to provide help and support for carers, including Princess Royal Trust for Carers, Crossroads Association and Carers UK (see help list).

Financial pressures

MS often affects people who are in the prime of their careers, with possible implications on their future earning capacity. If you have family, a mortgage and other commitments, financial concerns can be another major issue. Without the right support, this too can cause relationship problems.

It is important not to make any sudden decisions about employment or financial matters. Chapter 13 refers to these issues in more detail.

Usually, once children know that their parent is not going to die of MS and that nobody else in the family is likely to develop it, they can begin to accept it as part of family life.

Relationships with children

Bringing up children is challenging – with or without MS. It is easy to fall into the trap of blaming relationship problems with your children on the impact of MS in family life. In reality, most of these problems will be due to normal family issues.

Many parents worry about how and when to explain MS to their children. There is no right or wrong way of doing this, but it is important to recognise that children notice what goes on around them.

- Giving your child information about MS can stop it from becoming the 'monster in the wardrobe' and allows for questions to be asked and reassurances to be given.

- Usually, once children know that their parent is not going to die of MS and that nobody else in the family is likely to develop it, they can begin to accept it as part of family life.

- Teenagers bring many more dimensions to the situation, though exactly what sort of effects the addition of MS has in any individual family setting is difficult to work out.

- If you are finding these relationships increasingly difficult, it can help to seek informal advice from other parents in a similar situation through your local MS Society branch. You could also consult your GP about a possible referral for family therapy where all the members of the family could talk through the situation and consider ways forward.

- There are books and DVDs to help you speak to your child or teenager about MS available from the MS Society and the MS Trust (see help list).

Relationships with other family members

The impact of MS on relationships with extended family will depend on many factors, not least of which is their understanding of MS and how it affects you as an individual.

Parents of adult children with MS

Regardless of how old a child is when MS is diagnosed, parents might experience a whole host of emotions ranging from grief and anxiety to anger and guilt.

Fear can lead to 'guilt-ridden' behaviours, which can be eased if parents can find support and have the opportunity to express their concerns and ask questions of health professionals. It can help to seek advice and information from those in a similar situation through your local MS Society branch or through one of the organisations listed in the back of this book.

Extended family

We have previously looked at the 'unconscious' roles people play in their close relationships. This can include relationships with extended family. For example, if a sibling who has always been the 'organiser' is diagnosed with MS, they may have to reduce their commitments and delegate more in order to help manage their condition. It can take time for extended family members, who do not understand the day-to-day challenges of living with MS, to adjust to these changes. Information and communication are essential if misunderstandings are to be avoided.

Elderly relatives

MS is frequently diagnosed in young adulthood. There are many adults who have been living with MS for years and who have certain care needs of their own, but also find themselves acting as a carer for their elderly relatives.

One of the confusing aspects of MS is that it can upset the natural order of things. For example, a middle-aged person with MS might have assumed this caring role for their elderly relatives by virtue of the fact that they are younger in years. The irony is that although they may look physically younger, MS fatigue alone can some days make a person feel decades older than they really are.

Once a role such as this is established, it can be very difficult to ask for help without feeling you are letting your relatives down. Whilst you all appear to be coping, the situation is manageable, though far from ideal. If you have a relapse, there will be the additional worry of organising support for your relatives.

Your local social services department can advise you about services that may be needed now or later. Having a contingency plan can reduce anxiety about the future and enable you to concentrate on the present.

Friends and colleagues

It can be difficult for you to know what to say to friends and colleagues – most people don't understand it and even those who have come across it before may have formed the wrong perception of it.

- Many people in the early stages after diagnosis try to underplay any difficulties they are experiencing, particularly if they are caused by invisible symptoms referred to earlier in this book. The danger with this is that friends and colleagues will not understand when you are having a bad day and may misinterpret your behaviour or mood. This can escalate and lead to relationship problems.

- It is important for friends and colleagues to learn how MS can affect someone physically and emotionally in order for them to understand and adapt. But it is also important for them to appreciate that MS affects each person individually, that living with it is an ongoing learning curve for all affected, and that it must never be viewed by others as 'a convenient excuse' to avoid things.

- Some friendships can be harder to sustain – if, for example, a single shared interest becomes increasingly challenging for the person with MS. True friends will learn to adapt to changes in your circumstances.

- Many people with MS have found that it actually creates opportunities to meet people and get involved in things which would previously have seemed outside their comfort zone.

Young with MS

MS has historically been thought of as an adult condition, but it is now becoming apparent, although rare, that children and teenagers can also develop it.

- MS Society statistics indicate that between 5% and 10% of people diagnosed with MS will experience the onset before the age of 16.

- Young people face particular challenges living with a long-term condition. The publication, Childhood MS: A Guide for Parents covers the symptoms, diagnosis and treatment of childhood MS. It discusses what effects there can be on the child, the family and school life and explains the support available for parents and young people. It is available free from the MS Society (see help list).

- Teenagers and young adults with MS can often feel isolated and find it hard to make local contacts with others in a similar position. The Internet can be an excellent source of help if this is the case. Social networking sites where people can communicate informally without having to feel they are being labelled with MS are becoming increasingly popular.

Many people with MS have found that it actually creates opportunities to meet people and get involved in things which would previously have seemed outside their comfort zone.

- There are also excellent websites such as the MS Society's www.youngms.org.uk which has sections for both kids and teens.

Pregnancy and childbirth

MS is often diagnosed when people are in their 20s or 30s and are either thinking about starting a family or may have recently had a child. Pregnancy and childbirth is an area where misconceptions still abound.

Facts about pregnancy, childbirth and MS

- Pregnancy has no long-term effect on the course of MS and you are no more likely to experience miscarriage, stillbirth, birth defects or infant death than a woman who does not have MS.

- The chance of having a relapse actually goes down during pregnancy but increases in the first three months after delivery, before returning to the pre-pregnancy level.

- DMDs are not recommended for use during pregnancy, so it is important to discuss this specific issue with your GP, neurologist or MS nurse before you get pregnant.

- Breastfeeding does not alter the risk of relapses and there is no risk of passing on MS to your baby through breast milk, although use of DMDs by nursing mothers is not recommended.

Detailed information on this important subject is available from the MS Trust and the MS Society (see help list).

Summing Up

- Roles within relationships can alter, but one thing that MS does not change is the essence of who you are.

- Learning and practising good communication skills can help to deal with current and future conflicts.

- In a partnership or marriage where one person is classed as a 'carer', it is important for all to remember that this caring role is only one part of that relationship.

- The impact of MS on relationships with extended family will depend on many factors, not least of which is their understanding of MS and how it affects you as an individual.

- Communication is the key to maintaining healthy friendships.

- Statistics indicate that between 5% and 10% of people diagnosed with MS will experience the onset before the age of 16.

- Pregnancy has no long-term effect on the course of MS and you are no more likely to experience miscarriage, stillbirth, birth defects or infant death than a woman who does not have MS.

13

Practicalities

M S is frequently diagnosed when people are in the prime of their career and have family and financial commitments. It is important for you to know where to go for help and advice on a whole range of practical matters that might need addressing. This chapter deals with some of the common areas.

Meeting healthcare professionals

In addition to their primary role, health professionals can also be an essential link to other sources of information and external organisations. Making the best use of the time you get with them can lead to sources of help in many of the practical areas of life.

Many people diagnosed with MS will have little experience of the healthcare system and in the period after diagnosis it might feel as though the medical terminology associated with MS is a whole new language.

If you have been used to seeing your own GP, it can feel quite daunting to suddenly have a whole cross-section of health professionals involved in the management of your MS.

In time, you will see that because MS is such a complex and variable condition, all of these heath professionals are a much-needed part of a large jigsaw.

While your initial point of contact will usually be your GP or MS nurse, listed below are some of the other professionals that you may meet as part of a multidisciplinary health team:

Making the best use of the time you get with healthcare professionals can lead to sources of help in many of the practical areas of life.

- Neurologist: the neurologist is involved in the diagnostic procedure and in determining what medical treatment may be appropriate.

- Physiotherapist: physiotherapists are involved in the assessment of movement to help improve mobility. They can provide advice on exercise.

- Occupational therapist (OT): the main role of an OT is to assess your ability to perform daily activities and provide aids or adaptations, for example to help conserve energy and help with fatigue management.

- Continence advisor: this is a nurse who specialises in bladder and bowel problems. Their role is to assess the nature of any problem and provide advice on appropriate medication or other management strategies.

Depending on your individual MS symptoms and resulting health factors, you might also be seen at some stage by an ophthalmologist, pain specialist, dietician, psychologist or chiropodist.

Getting the most from your medical appointments

- Write down any questions you have before your appointment and take some paper so that you can make notes. It can also help to take somebody along with you who can jog your memory if needed.

- Try not to feel pressurised or rushed. Take your time and make sure that you get the most out of your appointment.

- If you disagree with your GP or neurologist, speak up! Your viewpoint is valid and you are the expert in your MS.

- Be honest with your doctors and specialists about your symptoms – tell them how you feel on bad days as well as good days.

Employment

People with MS can have a very strong work ethic and make very conscientious employees. A diagnosis of MS does not automatically take away the skills and experiences you have built up during years of employment.

However, the way someone is treated by their employer, along with the level of support and understanding they receive from colleagues following diagnosis, can have a significant impact on that individual's adjustment to living with MS.

In chapter 12 we looked at relationships and how a diagnosis of MS can act like a magnifying glass, showing up potential areas of conflict. Any pre-existing imbalance between your work and home life before MS can become harder to ignore as time goes on.

- It is important not to make any major decisions until you have got used to any changes and learnt more about managing your own MS.

- Most people with MS do continue to work for many years after receiving their diagnosis. This is more likely to happen if the employer has information about MS, including both physical and cognitive symptoms that might present challenges for you.

- Since 1995, people with MS have been covered by the Disability Discrimination Act (DDA) from the time of diagnosis – whether or not they are currently experiencing symptoms. Under the terms of this act, employers have a duty to consider making reasonable adjustments to make sure you are not put at substantial disadvantage by employment arrangements or physical features of the workplace.

The way someone is treated by their employer, along with the level of support and understanding they receive from colleagues following diagnosis, can have a significant impact on that individual's adjustment to living with MS.

What are reasonable adjustments?

These will vary according to resources available to your employer and would be considered only after consultation with the employee. They might include:

- Allocating some of your work to someone else.

- Transferring you to another post or another place of work.

- Considering whether some of the work could be done from home.

- Making adjustments to the buildings where you work, the furniture, equipment or tools that you use.

- Being flexible about your hours, allowing you to have different core working hours, and incorporating more breaks into your day.

Who needs to be told?

Under the DDA, you do not have to inform an employer about your MS unless you are in the armed forces or you work on a plane or ship. However, some employment contracts specifically request that you tell your employer and so it is important to check.

People with a driving licence who have been diagnosed with MS must tell the DVLA.

If your job requires you to drive, for example if you drive a heavy goods vehicle or passenger transport, you must inform your employer.

Where can I get information and support about employment?

Information is a key element here. Fortunately, there is no longer any reason for someone with MS to struggle on alone. There are many sources of help and information detailed in the help list at the back of this book, including:

- The MS Trust.
- The MS Society.
- Occupational therapists.
- Occupational health – in the workplace.
- Union representative.
- Disability employment advisor (DEA) at your local Jobcentre Plus.

Point of Diagnosis (www.pointofdiagnosis.org.uk) is a website with information on the DDA which protects people with MS from discrimination in the workplace, education, housing or in accessing services from the point of diagnosis.

Finances

Most people are diagnosed with MS when at the peak of their working lives, with young families and mortgages to maintain. At the same time as coming to terms with a diagnosis of a life-long condition, you may also have concerns about employment which can lead to anxiety about how the bills are to be paid.

This is a complex area and each person will have a different set of circumstances. The rules and regulations governing eligibility to pensions and benefits are also complicated and appear to change frequently, so it is not possible to give detailed advice within the context of this book.

- Many people find asking for help of this sort particularly difficult. This is normal. It can help to break things down into manageable steps – the first, and most important, is to gather as much information as possible. What you decide to do next with that information is a different step.

It can help to break things down into manageable steps – the first, and most important, is to gather as much information as possible.

- Do not be persuaded to pay for advice regarding benefits! The best people to contact for advice on your particular circumstances, and who can help you apply for any benefits you are eligible for, are your local Citizen's Advice Bureau or Welfare Rights Office. The MS Society may also have a local welfare rights adviser who can provide impartial advice. The key message with finances is not to struggle on alone until things have reached crisis point! (See help list for details).

- Negotiating the benefits system at the same time as learning to live with MS is not easy. Each time you recover from a relapse and begin to feel better, you may begin to doubt yourself, 'Will they think I'm making it up?'. Remember that benefit tribunals exist to prevent fraud, not to prevent you from obtaining benefits. When you fill in a benefit form, describe your worst days even if you are having a good spell.

- Find out what you are entitled to and claim it. Don't feel embarrassed about claiming, and never feel that you are being a 'scrounger'.

- If you are unable to go out without help, you may be entitled to free prescriptions.

When you have a condition like MS, your independence becomes even more important.

Insurance

Do I need to tell my insurance company?

If you are taking out a new insurance policy, you must always answer any questions honestly or the insurance will be invalid.

Before disclosing to existing insurers, it is best to check the policy booklet or seek advice from the MS Society helpline (see help list).

Mobility

When you have a condition like MS, your independence becomes even more important. If you are experiencing problems with your balance and walking ability, contact your GP or MS nurse. They will be able to arrange for an assessment by a physiotherapist or occupational therapist.

- A physiotherapist will assess you to see if there are any exercises, walking aids or other therapies which may help you get around more safely.

- An occupational therapist will look at the problems you have around the house and can arrange for various aids and adaptations which you may find useful.

Although it can be a very difficult decision to make, if you find that you are restricted in terms of where you can go and how long you can stay once you get there, it might be worth considering a wheelchair.

Case studies

'I see my wheelchair as a tool which enables me to get more out of life. A builder uses power tools to get a job done quicker and save energy; I use a wheelchair for the same reasons.' TM.

'I'm the same person in the wheelchair as I am out of it, and don't see any reason for people to talk to me any differently – although unfortunately there's still a lot of ignorance about. Well-meaning people can sometimes be quite patronising when I'm out and about with my wife. I can never understand why they seem to think that because I'm in a wheelchair I'm also deaf?' JC.

Many people with MS own a wheelchair which they keep under the stairs or in the boot of the car for occasional use only – to be used when they are having a bad day. In this way, you can stay in control of where and when you go out and manage your fatigue more effectively.

The Disabled Living Foundation, Assist UK and Remap are organisations that can provide information about equipment and adaptations (see help list).

If you have not already done so, it is a good idea to learn to drive. Some people only take lessons after they become disabled to avoid having to depend on others.

Driving

When you are diagnosed with MS, it is important that you notify both the DVLA and your insurance company in order to comply with law.

If you have not already done so, it is a good idea to learn to drive. Some people only take lessons after they become disabled to avoid having to depend on others.

If you are receiving the highest rate of the mobility component of the DLA, you can take advantage of the Motability scheme. This scheme enables disabled drivers to have a car adapted to their needs and is available to drivers and passengers alike.

The Blue Badge Scheme provides a range of parking concessions for people with severe mobility problems who have difficulty using public transport. For information about this scheme, visit www.direct.gov.uk.

Summing Up

- In addition to their main role, health professionals can be an essential link to other sources of information and external organisations. Making the best use of the time you get with them can also lead to help in many of the practical areas of life.

- The way someone is treated by their employer, along with the level of support and understanding they receive from colleagues following diagnosis, can have a significant impact on that individual's adjustment to living with MS.

- It is important that before making any decisions about continuing or leaving work, or about benefits and pensions, that you think them through carefully and after seeking free impartial advice.

- When you have a condition like MS, your independence becomes even more important, and with the right information you can take better control of this.

- When you are diagnosed with MS, it is important that you notify both the DVLA and your insurance company.

14

Living with MS

Taking control

MS is one condition where pushing yourself, rather than pacing yourself, is not helpful! It requires a change in mindset to how we are often conditioned to think by today's 24-hour society. It can also require a thick skin, and an understanding that unhelpful attitudes towards disability are often based on ignorance or misinformation; they are not personal.

There are many ways you can take back control of your life with MS including:

- Becoming your own expert – understand how your actions can affect your energy levels, so that you can plan your day and pace yourself.

- Find out about symptoms and how to cope with them.

- Make a 'relapse plan' when you are well so that you can look after yourself.

- If you feel you are having problems with memory and thinking, try giving yourself plenty of time, avoiding distractions, focusing on one thing at a time and planning ahead.

MS is one condition where pushing yourself, rather than pacing yourself is not helpful!

Most people with MS take an active interest in managing their health. In fact, after diagnosis, many people who have previously taken their health for granted begin to realise the benefits of regular sensible exercise, healthy heating and other measures such as complementary therapies.

In previous chapters, we talked about how MS can be like a magnifying glass, showing up potential problem areas that might add to the challenges you face. This same concept can apply to physical and emotional wellbeing.

Looking after your mind and body can be another way of taking back some control of your life alongside any conventional treatment regime you may have been prescribed.

With any of the strategies described in this chapter, it is important that you take time to find what works best for you, and always seek advice from health professionals before embarking on anything physically or emotionally demanding.

Staying active

Will exercise make my MS worse?

There is no evidence that exercise makes MS worse or that exercising causes relapses. In fact, studies at the University of Buffalo, USA, have shown that exercise can actually help those living with MS by building strength and endurance, reducing depression and increasing feel-good endorphins. It can also reduce risks caused through loss of muscle strength, weight problems and osteoporosis.

Which sort of exercise is best?

A physiotherapist can advise on exercises that meet specific needs and abilities – what suits one person will not suit another. These can include:

- Strengthening exercises – including lifting and moving small weights, or using the body's own weight to strengthen muscles and bones.
- Aerobic exercises – such as cycling, running or rowing.
- Stretching – helps keep muscles supple and relaxed.
- Range-of-motion – involves moving joints so that they go through as full a range of movement as possible.
- Passive stretching – involves a physiotherapist or carer helping to move your arms or legs to create a stretch and move the joints.
- Posture exercises – help keep your feet, knees, pelvis, shoulders and head properly aligned, to reduce strain on the muscles and bones in the body.
- Water-based exercise – strengthening, stretching and aerobic exercise can all be done in a pool. The water supports the body, lessening the stress placed on joints and muscles.

There are also various aids and adaptations that some people find useful with exercise, including:

- Ankle supports.
- Walking poles.
- Functional electrical stimulation (FES).
- Cooling devices.

Looking after your mind and body can be another way of taking back some control of your life alongside any conventional treatment regime you may have been prescribed.

Your MS nurse or other health professionals such as a physiotherapist or occupational therapist will be able to advise you about this.

If you have not exercised for a while, or are thinking of significantly increasing the amount you do, speak to your GP beforehand to be sure what you do is safe.

Some important points to remember:

- Listen to your body – some days you may be able to do more than others.
- Choose an activity you enjoy.
- Start slowly with any regime.
- Warm up and cool down.
- Heat sensitivity is common in MS and can make symptoms feel temporarily worse.
- Drink cool fluids and exercise in a well-ventilated space.

For further information about the benefits of exercise and physiotherapy in MS, ask your MS nurse or see the book list.

Diet and nutrition

If you have been diagnosed with MS, it might seem that on top of any other changes in your life, the last thing you want is advice about what you should eat and drink.

Conventional medications might treat relapses, symptoms or modify the course of your MS, but a well-balanced diet can help you maintain a healthy lifestyle, lessen fatigue and minimise the chance of getting infections.

It doesn't have to be restrictive, difficult or expensive to follow a balanced diet. The following general advice applies to all people – not just those with MS:

- Eat a wide variety of carbohydrates, fruit and vegetables, dairy products, meat, fish and alternatives, fat and sugar.
- Eat five portions of fruit and vegetables each day.
- Drink 8-10 cups (1-2 litres) of liquid a day, especially water.
- Eat high fibre foods.
- Grill, steam, bake or poach food instead of frying.

- Replace high fat or sugary foods with low fat/low sugar alternatives.
- Drink alcohol in moderation according to Department of Health guidelines.

Essential fatty acids

Essential fatty acids (EFAs) are polyunsaturated fats, such as linolenic acid and alpha linolenic acid. They play an important role in maintaining the central nervous system and the myelin sheath. Although there is no definitive evidence of long-term benefit, it makes sense to ensure a good intake of EFAs if you have MS.

- Linolenic acid is found in sunflower and soya oils, beans, peas and lentils and alpha linolenic acid in dark green, leafy vegetables, broccoli, green pepper and oily fish.
- Supplements rich in EFAs, such as evening primrose, starflower and wheat-germ oil are available over-the-counter, but can be expensive. You don't need to take special vitamin supplements if you eat a healthy and varied diet, but if you do take vitamins or supplements of any kind, make sure you do not exceed the recommended dose – there can be risks in taking large amounts.

Scientific studies are also taking place into the significance of antioxidants, B group vitamins, minerals and trace elements in MS.

Is there a special diet for MS?

Claims have been made about many diets said to help MS – low fat, gluten free, dairy free, etc. Studies so far have not provided conclusive scientific evidence of benefits.

- Some people find that following a restrictive diet is another way of helping them to feel like they're 'taking back some control' over their MS. It is important to seek advice from a GP or qualified dietician before following a restrictive diet, as some types of diets can actually be bad for your health.
- Tea, coffee and alcohol can all increase the need to pass urine, so avoid them if they cause problems.
- There is some evidence that a daily intake of 1-2 glasses of cranberry juice can help reduce urinary tract infections.
- Keeping a food and symptom diary for a while can help to identify foods you can and can't tolerate.

Complementary and alternative medicine are sometimes used alongside conventional healthcare and are accepted as complementing it, or as an alternative to it.

For further information about diet and nutrition in MS, ask your MS nurse or see the book list.

Complementary and alternative therapies

Complementary and alternative medicine are sometimes used alongside conventional healthcare and are accepted as complementing it, or as an alternative to it.

- Many people with MS report that complementary and alternative therapies help them to feel better. Although there is little research to show how effective or safe some of these medicines may be, the attitudes of conventional healthcare professionals towards these therapies is becoming more positive.

- Almost half of GP practices in England now provide access to some sort of complementary and alternative medicines for NHS patients.

- Check with your healthcare professionals before commencing any form of complementary therapy.

- It is important to do some background research and to find a properly trained and qualified practitioner.

Be prepared to try a range of treatments, but one at a time so that you can tell which therapy works for you. According to the MS Society, some of the therapies most commonly asked about by people with MS include:

- Acupuncture: a form of traditional Chinese medicine involving the insertion of thin, metallic needles by a trained practitioner in specific points of the body with the aim of improving energy flow.

- Acupressure: another form of traditional Chinese medicine involving the application of hand or finger pressure to specific points of the body with the aim of improving energy flow.

- Aromatherapy: a healing method that uses essential oils from plants which are either applied to the skin, mixed with bath water or inhaled.

- Homeopathy: a form of complementary medicine based on the principle of 'like cures like' by using miniscule amounts of a specific 'symptom-causing' substance with the aim of relieving that same symptom.

- Massage: a healing method that has been practiced for thousands of years which can be used on its own, or as one component of more broad-based healing methods such as aromatherapy.

- Pilates: a form of bodywork during which individuals focus on the use and control of specific muscles during body movements, with an emphasis on breathing.

- Reflexology: uses the application of pressure to specific areas, or zones, on the foot with the aim of improving health by increasing energy flow in the body.

- Relaxation and meditation: uses a number of techniques including imagery and progressive muscle relaxation and is believed to reduce stress and anxiety and encourage a more positive outlook.

- T'ai chi: a traditional Chinese martial art using sequences of body postures connected by slow, graceful movements. It is believed to have a number of benefits including improved muscle stiffness, vitality and social and emotional functioning.

- Yoga: a mind-body therapy that uses a combination of breathing, meditation and posture in order to promote physical and emotional wellbeing.

Once you are better informed, you can then sift through that knowledge to find what works best for you.

Other well-known complementary and alternative therapies include: chiropractic medicine, healing, herbal medicine, multi-modal therapy, osteopathy, reiki, shiatsu, toning tables. Detailed information about these can be obtained from publications in the book list supplied at the end of this book.

'Non-standard' therapies

There are a number of non-standard therapies that people claim have helped their MS symptoms, but the benefits claimed are as yet unproven by large scale clinical studies and unknown risks can also be involved.

- Cannabis and cannabis extracts: these contain cannabinoids which have a variety of biological effects. People with MS have suggested that cannabis may alleviate symptoms including spasticity and pain. Further studies of the effects of cannabis are planned in the UK.

- Cooling: a complementary therapy unique to MS which is reported to improve certain symptoms. It can involve simple methods such as staying in air-conditioned areas and drinking cold liquids, or more complex techniques using specially designed cooling suits.

- Honey bee venom: a type of therapy called apitherapy which refers to the use of bees or bee products to treat medical conditions. Studies have yet to prove significant beneficial effects in people with MS.

- Hyperbaric oxygen therapy: a form of treatment in which oxygen is administered under increased pressure in a specially designed chamber in order to increase the oxygen content in blood and body tissues. Studies have yet to confirm any proven beneficial effect in people with MS.

Other non-standard therapies can include: magnetic field therapy, neural therapy, replacement of mercury amalgam fillings, transcutaneous nerve stimulation (TENS). Detailed information about these can be obtained from publications in the book list supplied at the end of this book.

There is a lot of information available about complementary and alternative medicines. The problem, particularly when looking on the Internet, is finding information that is objective and accurate. Anyone can publish a website without needing to supply names, qualifications or sources, and even without checking the information is based on scientific research.

Always consult with your healthcare professionals before making any decisions about complementary or alternative therapies. Where possible, consult a practitioner who has been personally recommended to you (by a friend, health food store, GP) and always tell your practitioner that you have MS.

Detailed information about complementary and alternative therapies can be obtained through the MS Society and MS Trust (see help list).

Many people are surprised to find that although MS can sometimes make them feel "different" to their circle of family and friends, it can expand and enrich their social circle.

Staying informed and supported

Although a person's reaction to a diagnosis of MS can be as varied and unpredictable as the condition itself, it's important to remember that there is a wealth of information and support available, including a wide range of practical and emotional coping strategies which were not there 20 years ago.

This progress is continuing even as this book goes to print. If you would like to take a proactive role in managing your MS, it is a good idea to stay informed through reliable sources.

It can save time, energy and even money to find out about some of these ideas and strategies through the organisations referred to in this book instead of struggling on alone, or learning the hard way.

Once you are better informed, you can then sift through that knowledge to find what works best for you.

Never allow others to fob you off if they can't immediately provide the information you need, but be prepared to do your own research too and try to keep up-to-date with the latest findings through the following:

- MS organisations such as the MS Society and the MS Trust.

- MS nurses and MS therapy centres.

- Courses for the newly diagnosed.

- Living with long-term conditions courses.

In the help list you will find contact information for MS organisations and other useful organisations.

An expanding circle

It is understandable after diagnosis to feel a sense of isolation and perhaps want to avoid seeing or hearing anything to do with MS. This is natural. The condition is only one part of your life and you don't want to become defined by it. Despite this, many people are surprised to find that although MS can sometimes make them feel 'different' to their circle of family and friends, it can also expand and enrich their social circle.

It can be really helpful to talk to other people with MS, either face to face, on the phone or over the Internet. The MS Society has a network of branches all over the country including members and volunteers of all ages and from all backgrounds.

If you have access to the Internet, you may prefer to join a chat room or forum. The MS Trust runs regular chat rooms on different topics related to MS and these are supported by a range of relevant health professionals.

Case study

'I have been enjoying reflexology treatments every few weeks for about three years now. Each session lasts about 40 minutes. I have found the main benefit to be increased energy levels in addition to fewer cramping sensations in my legs – especially during a relapse.' JM.

Summing Up

- It is important that you take time to find what works best for you, and always seek advice from health professionals before embarking on anything physically or emotionally demanding.

- There is no evidence that exercise makes MS worse, or that exercising causes relapses. In fact, studies have shown that exercise can actually help those living with MS to manage their symptoms.

- A well-balanced diet can help you maintain a healthy lifestyle, lessen fatigue and minimise the chance of getting infections.

- Complementary and alternative medicine are sometimes used alongside conventional healthcare and accepted as complementing it, or as an alternative to it.

- Never allow others to fob you off if they can't immediately provide the information you need, but be prepared to do your own research too and try to keep up-to-date with the latest findings through reliable sources.

- Many people are surprised to find that although having MS can sometimes make them feel 'different' to their circle of family and friends, it can also expand and enrich that circle.

Help List

Ability Net

Tel: 0800 269 545
Contact form: https://www.abilitynet.org.uk/how-contact-us
Website: https://www.abilitynet.org.uk/
Info: Offers advice, support, assessment of needs and the supply of adapted computer equipment for people with any sort of disability.

Carers Trust

Address: Carers Trust, 32-36 Loman Street, London SE1 0EH
Tel: 0300 772 9600
Email: info@carers.org
Website: https://carers.org/
Info: Carers Trust is the leading charity helping carers in the UK.

Disability, Pregnancy & Parenthood

Address: National Centre for Disabled Parents, Unit F9, 89-93 Fonthill Road, London, N4 3JH
Tel: 0800 018 4730
Contact form: http://disabledparent.org.uk/contact-us
Website: http://disabledparent.org.uk/
Info: Promotes better awareness and support for disabled people during pregnancy and as parents.

Disabled Living Foundation

Address: Disabled Living Foundation, Unit 1, 34 Chatfield Road, Wandsworth, London SW11 3SE
Tel: 0300 999 0004
Email: info@dlf.org.uk
Website: http://www.dlf.org.uk/
Info: Provides information on disability equipment, day-to-day household gadgets, new technologies and training techniques.

Disability Rights UK

Address: Ground Floor, CAN Mezzanine, 49-51 East Rd, London, N1 6AH

Tel: 020 7250 8181 (Not an advice line)

Email: enquiries@disabilityrightsuk.org

Website: https://www.disabilityrightsuk.org/

Info: UK charity advocating for the disabled, with the aim of creating a society where everyone can participate easily.

Jooly's Joint

Contact form: http://www.mswebpals.org/comment.htm

Website: http://www.mswebpals.org/

Info: An online community of people who live with MS. Has a special section for finding penpals with MS.

MS International Federation

Address: MS International Federation, Skyline House, 200 Union Street, London, SE1 0LX

Tel: 020 7620 1911

Contact form: https://www.msif.org/contact-us/

Website: https://www.msif.org/

Info: Includes links to national societies around the world and news of developments in MS research.

MS People UK

Website: http://www.ms-people.com/

Info: A forum for those with MS to share their experiences with the condition.

MS Society

Address: MS Society, MS National Centre (MSNC), 372 Edgware Road, London, NW2 6ND

Tel: 0808 800 8000

Email: supportercare@mssociety.org.uk

Website: https://www.mssociety.org.uk/

Info: Funds research, runs holiday homes and respite care, provides grants, education, information and training for people affected by MS.

MS Trust

Address: Spirella Building, Bridge Road, Letchworth Garden City, SG6 4ET

Tel: 0800 032 3839

Email: info@mstrust.org.uk

Website: https://www.mstrust.org.uk

Info: Provides information for anyone affected by MS, and has a map of MS services here: https://www.mstrust.org.uk/understanding-ms/who-can-help/map-ms-services

MS Trust: Staying Smart

Address: Spirella Building, Bridge Road, Letchworth Garden City, SG6 4ET

Tel: 0800 032 3839

Email: info@mstrust.org.uk

Website: http://www.stayingsmart.org.uk/

Info: Staying Smart is an online project from The MS Trust and Royal Holloway, University of London. Provides information about cognitive difficulties that may be experienced by people affected by MS.

Motability UK

Address: Motability Operations Ltd, City Gate House, 22 Southwark Bridge Road, London, SE1 9HB

Tel: 0300 456 4566

Contact form: https://www.motability.co.uk/contact-and-support/contact-information/general-enquiry-form

Website: http://www.motability.co.uk/

Info: A national UK charity which helps disabled people and their families to become more mobile.

Multiple Sclerosis National Therapy Centres

Address: MS National Therapy Centres, PO Box 2199, Buckingham, MK18 8AR

Tel: 01296 711699

Email: info@msntc.org.uk

Website: http://www.msntc.org.uk/

Info: Represents more than 70 self-help centres across England, Wales and Northern Ireland, providing a wide range of drug-free symptom management therapies.

Revive MS Support

Address: Revive MS Support, Moorpark Court, 29 Dava Street, Govan, Glasgow, G51 2JA
Tel: 0141 945 3344
Email: info@revivemssupport.org.uk
Website: https://www.revivemssupport.org.uk/
Info: Charity helping people affected by MS at every stage from diagnosis onwards, in particular in Scotland.

The Neurological Alliance

Address: Parkinson's UK, 215 Vauxhall Bridge Road, SW1V 1EJ
Tel: 020 7963 3994
Website: http://www.neural.org.uk/
Info: Enables charities to work together to improve quality of life for all those living in the UK with a neurological condition.

Book List

Coping with Multiple Sclerosis : A Comprehensive Guide to the Symptoms and Treatments
By Cynthia Benz, Ebury Publishing, London UK, 2005.

Everyday Health and Fitness with Multiple Sclerosis
By David Lyons, Fair Winds Press, Rockport USA, 2017.

Managing Multiple Sclerosis Naturally : A Self Help Guide to Living with MS
By Judy Graham, Inner Traditions Bear and Company, Rochester USA, 2010.

Multiple Sclerosis for Dummies
By Rosalind Kalb, John Wiley & Sons, NY USA, 2012.

Multiple Sclerosis : New Hope and Practical Advice for People with MS and Their Families
By Louis J. Rosner, Fireside Books, NY USA, 2008.

Multiple Sclerosis (Oxford Neurology Library)
By Neil Scolding, OUP, Oxford UK, 2012.

Multiple Sclerosis : The Facts You Need
By Paul O'Connor, Firefly Books, Ontario Canada, 1999.

Multiple Sclerosis : Understanding the Cognitive Challenges
By Nicholas LaRocca, Demos Medical Publishing, NY USA, 2006.

The "Everything" Health Guide to Multiple Sclerosis
By Margot Russel, Adams Media Corp., Holbrook MA USA, 2009.

Women Living with Multiple Sclerosis : Conversations on Living, Laughing and Coping
By Judity Lynn Nichols, Hunter House, Alameda CA USA, 1999.

Bibliography

Compston A, *et al.*, *McAlpine's Multiple Sclerosis (4th ed.),* Churchill Livingstone, London, 2005.

Disease modifying drug therapy – what you need to know, MS Trust, Letchworth, 2009, (available for free from www.mstrust.org.uk/publications).

Minden, S, 'Treatment of mood and affective disorders', in Ruddick, K and Goodkin D (eds), *Multiple Sclerosis Therapeutics*, Taylor and Francis, London, 1999.

MS Essentials 14: Fatigue, MS Society, London, 2008, (available for free from www.mssociety.org.uk/publications).

MS Essentials 18: Complementary and Alternative Medicine, MS Society, London, 2008, (available for free from www.mssociety.org.uk/publications).

MS Essentials 21: Exercise and Physiotherapy, MS Society, London, 2009, (available for free from www.mssociety.org.uk/publications).

MS Essentials 28: Living with the Effects of MS, MS Society, London, 2009, (available for free from www.mssociety.org.uk/publications).

MS: What Does It Mean for Me? A Positive and Practical Introduction to MS, MS Trust, Letchworth, 2007, (available for free from www.mstrust.org.uk/publications).

Rog, D, Burgess, M, Mottershead, J and Talbot, P, *Multiple Sclerosis: Answers at your fingertips (2nd ed.),* Class Publishing, London, 2009.

Sadovnick AD, *et al.,* 'A population- based study of multiple sclerosis in twins: update', *Annals of Neurology*, 1993, vol. 33, pages 281-85.

Schwid, S and Murray, TJ, 'Treating fatigue in patients with MS: one step forward, one step back', *Neurology*, 2005, vol. 64, pages 1111-2.

Swank, RL and Dugan, BB, 'Effects of Low Saturated Fat Diets in Early and Late Cases of MS', *The Lancet*, 1990, vol. 336, pages 27-39.

Tips for Living with MS, MS Trust, Letchworth, 2008, (available for free from www.mstrust.org.uk/publications).